Reimagine Well Learn Guide:

Oncofertility

Fertility Preservation Options And Cancer

Martin Casella

Roger Holzberg

Adele Sender

"When I see a newly diagnosed oncofertility patient and meet with their family, one of the most important things that I want to get across in our first meeting is that they have choices. And that many of these choices were not available even five years ago."
— *Laxmi Kondapalli, M.D., MSCE*

"Always ask about the impact of treatment on fertility as a part of informed consent before cancer treatment starts."
— *Julie Messina, PA-C*

This Oncofertility Learn Guide is designed to help patients and their families overcome the fear and anxiety of a cancer diagnosis, and to educate them on the Fertility Preservation issues that may result from treatment.

Our goal is to provide concise, evidence-based, easily understood resources to be used throughout the entire cancer journey and to provide a (private and safe) support community where patients and their families can learn from survivors and caregivers who have already been on this journey.

—Team Reimagine Well

TABLE OF CONTENTS

NOTE:

Both Parts 1 and 2 of this Learn Guide are designed to go hand in hand. We strongly encourage you to read forward only to the phase you are in at this moment:

- Diagnosis
- Healing
- Treatment
- Wellbeing

As you use Part 1 to educate yourself - and get coached on how to become an empowered patient - you may want to create your online patient or caregiver Support Community, which can be accessed at http://www.reimaginewellcommunity.com/reimaginewell. The details on how to best use the Support Community are found in Part 2 of this Learn Guide.

Three messages to newly diagnosed patients (and your families,) who have concerns about your reproductive future.

From Leonard Sender, M.D., Co-Founder of Reimagine Well.

"Information can lead to knowledge. Knowledge is power. You have to become empowered to learn, then ask the right questions and get the information you need. The best way to get the type of treatment that is right for you, that will lead to the type of outcome we want for you, is to become fully engaged in the process."

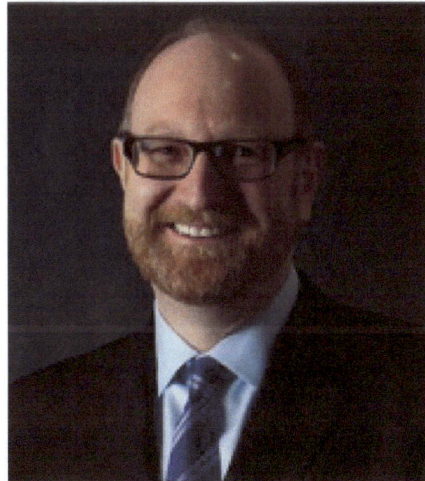

The following messages are from Julia Messina, PA-C, and Laxmi Kondapalli, M.D. Both are experts in the medical field of Oncofertility.

"Patients with cancer and their families need to start thinking about fertility preservation at the time of the patient's diagnosis. There may be several options available to a patient, but many of these options must be performed before cancer treatment begins."
— *Julie Messina, PA-C*

"My role as an oncofertility specialist is to not only think about the fertility issues of my patients, but also to expand that to consider the whole host of long-term reproductive side effects that may result as an outcome of cancer treatment."
— *Laxmi Kondapalli, M.D., MSCE*

Have a copy of this Enhanced eBook with you at all meetings with your Health Team and Healthcare Professionals, and use it as a guide to get all of your pre-treatment questions answered.

— Team Reimagine Well

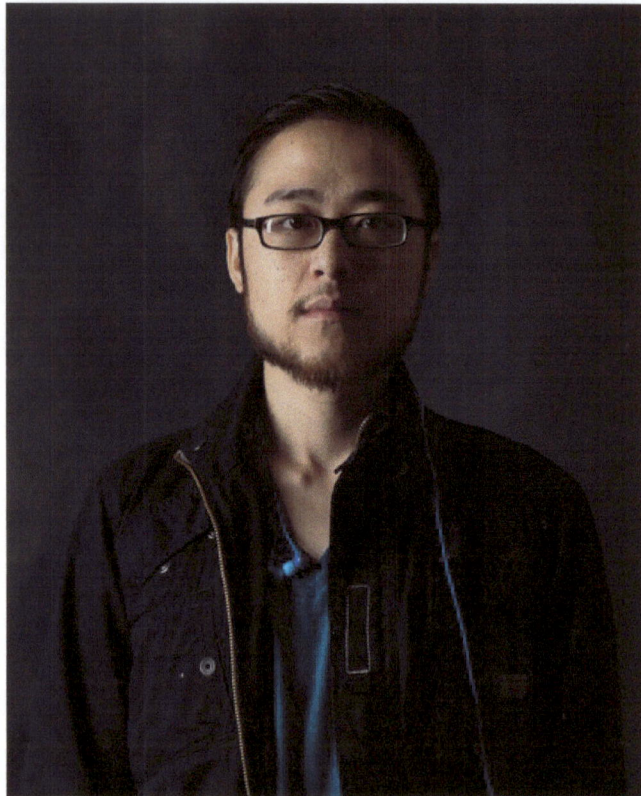

CONTRIBUTING EXPERTS

4

Dr. Kondapalli is board certified in Obstetrics and Gynecology and the subspecialty Reproductive Endocrinology and Infertility, and is a Fellow of the American Congress of Obstetricians and Gynecologists.

Her research interests center on fertility preservation, ovarian response to medical therapies, and assisted reproduction outcomes. She has authored many publications in the area of reproductive medicine, serves on the scientific advisory boards of multiple oncology groups, and was the recipient of the 2013 AAMC Women in Medicine and Science Professional Leadership Award. At the time this Oncofertility guide was created, she was on faculty at the University of Colorado as Assistant Professor in the Division of Reproductive Endocrinology and Infertility, and recipient of a National Institutes of Health Career Development grant.

She is currently a physician at the Colorado Center for Reproductive Medicine.

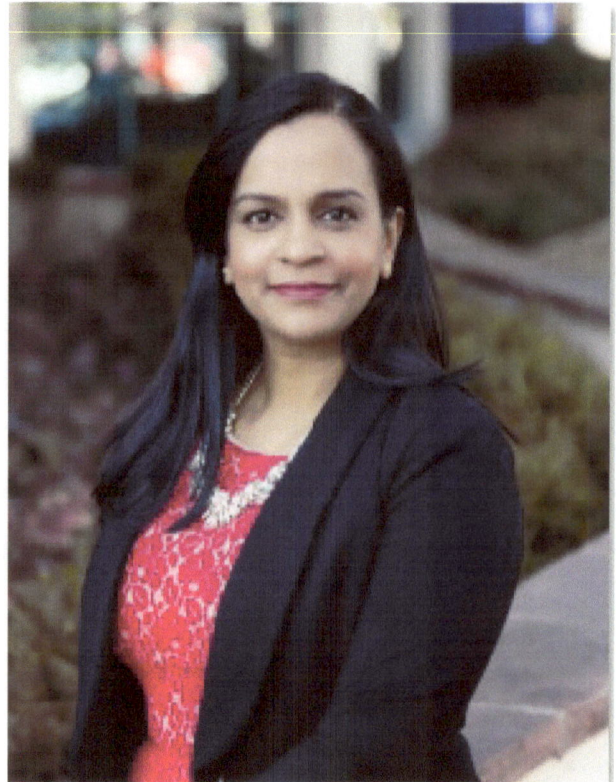

Laxmi Kondapalli, M.D., MSCE

"I would describe myself as a physician/ scientist. I see patients in a clinical setting, and I do a lot of research looking closely at clinical outcomes."

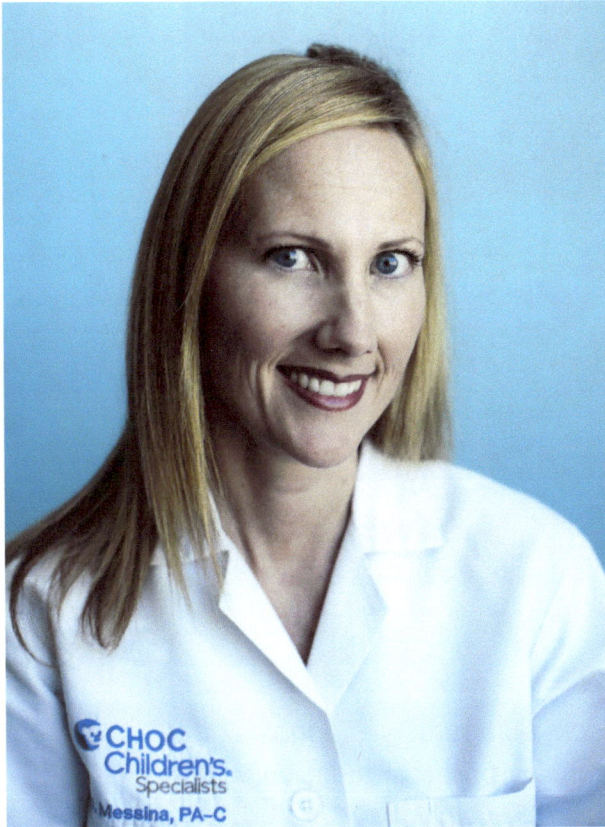

Julie Messina, PA-C, is a licensed Physician Assistant in the field of Oncology. Julie was inspired to work in this field by her experience with young adult patients during their Survivorship, in the hope of giving them the most meaningful lives beyond cancer. She currently lives in Colorado with her husband and son, and enjoys skiing and white water rafting.

Julie Messina, Physician Assistant

"My name is Julie Messina. I work as a part of the team with cancer doctors. We're thinking about the long-term consequences, about things we can do to help children have a very long healthy life beyond their treatment."

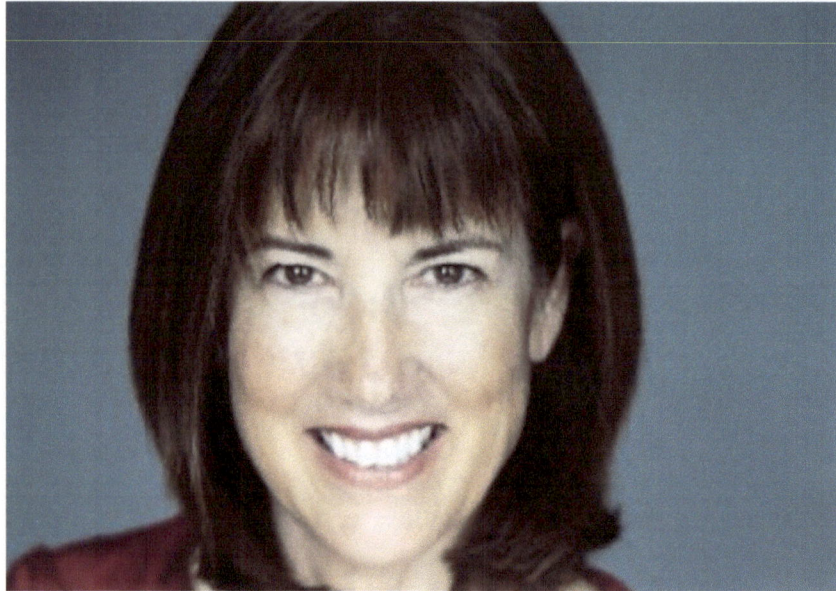

Jocelyn Harrison, MPH, RD

"My name is Jocelyn Harrison. Although a diagnosis can be overwhelming, you have a part to play in your own treatment. Be empowered. This is your journey."

Jocelyn Harrison received her Master of Public Health from UCLA and completed a dietetic internship at the Los Angeles Veterans Hospital. She has developed nutrition programs and marketing for the USDA Dietary Guidelines for Americans, Choose Health LA, and the American Diabetes Association. In addition to nutritional and lifestyle advice, her Reimagine Well work includes literature reviews and helping with "immersive healing environment" patient benefit studies.

"You're stronger than you think. I wish you all the best on your oncofertility journey!"

— Julie Messina, PA-C

Oncofertility is a relatively new medical field, combining oncology (the specialized study of cancer, its diagnosis, and treatment) with research into how the human reproductive system is affected by cancer. The actual term oncofertility was created in 2006 by Dr. Teresa K. Woodruff of The Oncofertility Consortium, and is now officially recognized as the term for cancer fertility preservation in the English language.

Beginning as a study into the clinical care of women who are at risk of losing their fertility due to cancer treatment, oncofertility has since grown to incorporate men's fertility issues, along with other post-cancer treatment reproductive challenges, such as family planning, complex contraception, safety of pregnancy, surrogacy, adoption and hormonal management throughout survivorship.

Those who study and work in oncofertility are continually exploring and expanding the options for the reproductive future of cancer survivors. The Oncofertility Consortium itself can be a wonderful research source on your oncofertility journey, as you'll learn below.

Why oncofertility is important to you, and what you need to know RIGHT NOW, is that for many recently diagnosed cancer patients - whether male or female, and depending on the type of cancer therapy prescribed - your treatment can seriously damage or even destroy your ability to father a child if you're male, or to conceive, carry and give birth to a child if you're female. So while you are dealing with the shock and complexity of a cancer diagnosis, and trying to understand treatment options and a whole new vocabulary, you also need to be thinking about what you can do to preserve your future fertility.

Oncofertility is a significant issue for cancer patients of all ages, as well as family members and caregivers. For cancer patients in their teens, young adulthood, and early middle age, the reality of not being able to have children can be a heartbreaking experience. For recently diagnosed patients, an immediate consultation to discuss fertility preservation by an oncofertility specialist is absolutely crucial.

The concept and practice of oncofertility has, for many cancer patients, greatly improved the opportunities to become parents. Our Reimagine Well expert, Julie Messina, who is a Physician's Assistant in the field of Oncofertility, believes patients should seek out hospitals where the staff is "educated and constantly thinking about fertility preservation for their patients." If you need help finding a hospital or medical center with such a staff, contact The Oncofertility Consortium or visit their website at http://oncofertility.northwestern.edu/.

"The sperm can be protected - even on that day of diagnosis - until that time when the patient might need it, somewhere down the line, for their own fertility."

— *Teresa Woodruff, Ph.D*

In today's medical world, those who've made it through their cancer journey are looking forward to a future of long-term survivorship due to improved cancer treatments.

However, many of those therapies that have so effectively increased survival rates also have serious side effects that also may cause the loss of fertility much later in life.

Another of our Reimagine Well experts, Dr. Laxmi Kondapalli, not only treats recently diagnosed cancer patients for their immediate fertility preservation challenges, but also helps them deal with these later side effects that may affect their reproductive health.

"Fertility is one of the most important quality of life issues for many patients, especially those who are of reproductive age."
— *Laxmi Kondapalli, M.D., MSCE*

At Reimagine Well, we know that whether you are a patient, a member of the patient's family, or on their Care Team, you are under a tremendous amount of pressure right now.

You are not only at the beginning of your cancer journey, but your oncofertility journey as well.

You may be in a situation where you have to make some big decisions, very quickly.

You have a lot going on in your life. You may be overwhelmed. <u>That is completely normal.</u>

"Not to be able to have kids changes everything. So, you know, it's huge!"
— *20-Year-Old With Anaplastic Cell Lymphoma*

But it is crucial - for all of you - to understand the impact cancer treatment can have on reproductive health, especially for pediatric, adolescent and young adult patients.

What's at stake is not only your life, but your future ability to create life. Our goal is to quickly give you the educational background you need to make those decisions.

This is where we ask you - whether you are the patient, parent, caregiver, or a medical professional on the patient's Care Team - to stop and take a breath.

Then let it out. And remember… keep breathing.

There's one other thing you need to know before you continue onto the Learn Guide. You're not alone. Your family and friends are here. Your medical Care Team is here. And in case you missed the information earlier, there is another resource you have.

That is Reimagine Well's online Support Community. It's free, it's private and it's safe. You can meet others there who are going through the same thing you are. You'll also find cancer survivors who will share their experiences with you. That Community can be accessed online at http://www.reimaginewellcommunity.com/reimaginewell

AND PLEASE NOTE: Throughout the Learn Guide, there are videos available to watch if you prefer to do that. Here's the first one:

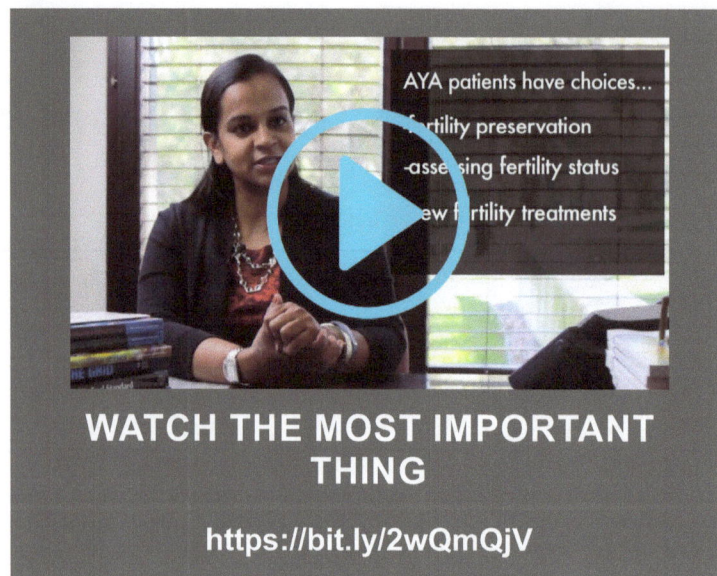

AYA patients have choices…
-fertility preservation
-assessing fertility status
-new fertility treatments

WATCH THE MOST IMPORTANT THING

https://bit.ly/2wQmQjV

TO LEARN MORE

Oncofertility: https://medlineplus.gov/magazine/issues/fall14/articles/fall14pg18-19.html
The Oncofertility Consortium: http://oncofertility.northwestern.edu

PART ONE: A "NEW NORMAL"

Notes

Diagnosis

Take A Deep Breath

What Now?

You've received your diagnosis. Your world is a little upside down right now. Soon, you, your family, and your Care Team will assemble to discuss various treatment options.

You know, from the introduction to this Oncofertility Learn Guide, that at this stage of your cancer journey a conversation with your oncologist about fertility preservation is extremely important.

It's important, because as you also know, some of the treatments cancer patients receive - both men and women - may actually impair their ability to have children in the future.

So - whether you are male or female - you **must** talk to your doctor now to see if there are fertility preservation options for you **BEFORE** you start your treatment. This will really optimize your options after the treatment phase.

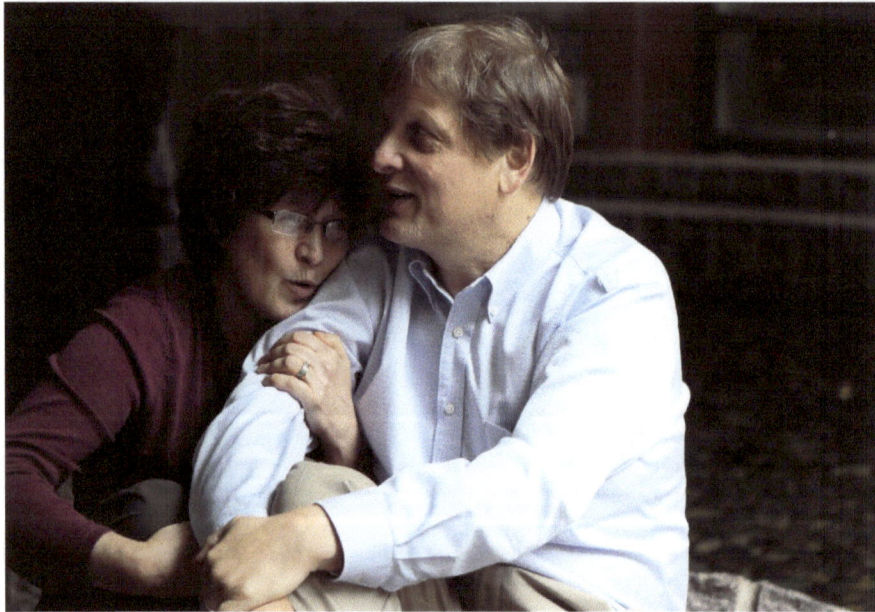

But first, in advance of meeting with your oncologist, let's learn just how your treatments can affect your fertility, and what fertility options you have before those treatments begin.

"We're thinking about the long-term consequences of the cure. We're thinking about things we can do to make sure patients have a long, healthy life beyond their treatment.
— *Julie Messina, PA-C*

How Different Cancer Treatments Affect Fertility

"Information is your friend. Ask lots of questions. Do lots of research!"
— *17-Year-Old With Lymphoma*

The first and foremost piece of information you need to know is that the reproductive health and fertility of men and women is affected in different ways by various cancer therapies.

That's why your oncologist and members of your Care Team need to explore all of the fertility preservation options when deciding which cancer treatment is right for you. Simply put, if you are a woman, your cancer - along with your cancer treatments, their side effects, and your fertility preservation options - will differ from a man's. And guys, vice versa for you.

"I love discussing fertility preservation with patients because it means that we are planning for their life beyond cancer. It is seen as a discussion of hope. I know that it will be important to them one day. Although there are many ways to make a family, I want my patients to someday have the option of biological children if they choose."
— *Julie Messina, PA-C*

Cancer Treatment Issues For Girls and Women

Females are born with all the eggs they will ever have. Cancer treatment can affect female patients by causing ovarian damage or failure, early menopause, genetic damage to growing eggs and other reproductive problems. There are particular cancer therapies that put women's reproduction at more risk. These include the following:

Chemotherapy kills rapidly-dividing cells in the body, targeting both cancerous cells and healthy ones. This can damage or destroy a female's eggs. Age, type of chemotherapy, and the medication dosage can impart various levels of risk. Particularly dangerous are those treatments using high doses of drugs referred to as alkylating agents. There is also the risk a young woman's ovaries will stop working (also known as primary ovarian insufficiency or premature menopause) with the use of certain cancer drugs. See the "Here's The Science" section following Part 1 of this guide for more information.

Radiation kills rapidly dividing cells in and around the target area at which the radiation is directed. When directed at or near the pelvic area, radiation can damage the reproductive system. Radiation to the hormone-producing areas of the brain or the pituitary gland may also cause infertility by disrupting normal hormone production. Direction of the radiation, and the dose, impacts the risk level. Since the human oocyte (an egg cell) is very sensitive to radiation, pelvic radiotherapy is also known to cause premature menopause. In addition, direct pelvic radiation may impair a woman's ability to carry a safe pregnancy. See "Here's The Science" for more information.

Bone Marrow/Stem Cell Transplant involves high doses of chemotherapy, and sometimes full body radiation. This poses a high infertility risk by damaging ovarian and uterine reproductive systems. In some cases, the damage may even eliminate future chances of carrying a pregnancy, depending on the amount and intensity of treatment.

Cancer Treatment Medications that specifically target cancer proteins can affect fertility. Medications that target other cancer characteristics appear to have limited effect on female fertility, but can impact the pregnancy itself.

Surgery can remove gynecologic cancers that have been found in a woman's reproductive system, such as ovarian, uterine, or cervical cancer. Removing the uterus, ovaries, cervix, or Fallopian tubes can cause infertility and/or eliminate chances of carrying a pregnancy.

In addition, any of these treatments can also have another specific consequence for female cancer patients. A woman's natural fertility declines over time, even outside of a cancer diagnosis. So when you add this natural decline in fertility to a woman's cancer treatments, the combination may actually accelerate that decline. This can mean that by the time a female patient has completed her cancer treatment, her fertility might be substantially reduced. That patient may even become infertile, and unable to have biological children of her own.

TO LEARN MORE

Fertility and Women With Cancer: https://bit.ly/2yf5w9P

About Chemotherapy: https://www.cancer.gov/about-cancer/treatment/types/chemotherapy

Premature ovarian insufficiency: https://www.medicinenet.com/premature_ovarian_failure_pof/article.html

About Radiation: https://www.cancer.gov/about-cancer/treatment/types/radiation-therapy

Bone Marrow/Stem Cell Transplant: https://bit.ly/2Psix6x

Cancer Treatment Medications That Specifically Target Cancer Proteins: https://www.cancer.gov/about-cancer/treatment/drugs

Fertility Options Available For Girls and Women

Post-pubertal girls and women (those who are menstruating) already have mature eggs in their ovaries, so they potentially have the option of freezing eggs, embryos and ovarian tissue.

Prepubescent girls (those who are not yet menstruating) have not yet produced mature eggs, so they are candidates for ovarian tissue cryopreservation. After cancer treatment, the ovarian tissue can be transplanted back into a patient's body.

Please note: The **ovarian tissue transplant** procedure is currently experimental, but has produced encouraging results in the past. However, ovarian tissue transplants are a very challenging area. Many diseases, such as leukemia, cause malignant cells to invade the ovaries. So preserving ovarian tissue with a plan to re-implant it one day raises the risk of reintroducing cancer to the patient. Scientists are investigating strategies to eliminate these malignant (cancerous) cells from a girl's ovarian tissue.

TO LEARN MORE

Fertility Preservation and Options for Women Starting Cancer Treatment: https://bit.ly/2PviJC8

The First Birth from Transplanted Tissue: http://www.popsci.com/woman-transplanted-ovarian-tissue-gives-birth-baby

Cancer Treatment Issues For Boys and Men

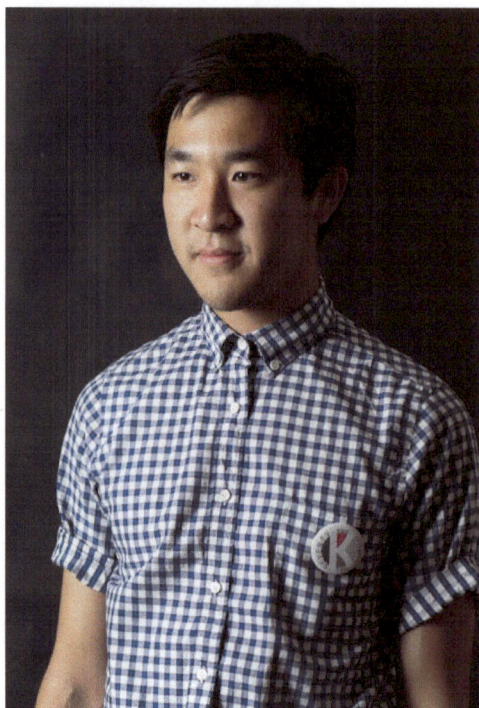

Cancer treatment can affect male patients by causing damage to the testes and interfering with sperm production. There are some treatments that put males more at risk. These include:

Chemotherapy kills rapidly-dividing cells in the body. This targets cancerous cells, but kills healthy ones as well. Some chemotherapy treatments are more harmful than others, particularly those using high doses of drugs referred to as alkylating agents. A male's age, the type of chemotherapy, and the drug dosage can influence a fertility risk.

Radiation kills rapidly dividing cells in and around the target area at which the radiation is directed. Radiation directed at or near the testicles can genetically damage a man's sperm or cause infertility. Radiation to the hormone-producing areas of the brain or the pituitary gland may also cause infertility by disrupting normal hormone production.

Bone Marrow/Stem Cell Transplant involves high doses of chemotherapy, and sometimes full body radiation. The combination of treatments and their intensity put the patient at a high risk for infertility.

Cancer Treatment Medications that specifically target cancer proteins can affect fertility. Medications that target other cancer characteristics appear to have limited effect on male fertility.

Surgery removes cancer-ridden parts of the body. Infertility can result when parts of the reproductive system – such as one or both testicles – are removed.

TO LEARN MORE

Fertility and Men with Cancer: https://bit.ly/2PEt52J

Chemotherapy: https://www.cancer.gov/about-cancer/treatment/types/chemotherapy

Radiation: https://www.cancer.gov/about-cancer/treatment/types/radiation-therapy

Bone Marrow/Stem Cell Transplant: https://bit.ly/2Psix6x

Cancer Treatment Medications That Specifically Target Cancer Proteins: https://www.cancer.gov/about-cancer/treatment/drugs

Fertility Options Available For Boys and Men

For **post-pubertal boys** (those who have gone through puberty) and men already producing sperm, the easiest and most mainstream fertility preservation method is sperm cryopreservation. Also known as sperm banking, this is a process where the patient's sperm is collected or harvested, and frozen for future use.

For prepubescent boys (those who have not yet gone through puberty, so they are not yet producing sperm), medical researchers are studying the best ways to freeze, store and use boys' testicular tissue to restore fertility in the future.

Please note: All males have three important cells in the testicles: the sertoli cell, which helps in sperm production; the leydig cell, which makes testosterone; and the spermatogonial stem cell, which also makes sperm. As long as the stem cell isn't damaged by cancer therapy, a post-pubertal patient can make sperm after completing cancer treatment. For prepubescent boys, since that stem cell is not creating sperm, sperm cannot yet be collected. New research is now focused on taking testicular biopsies to preserve the stem cell tissues.

TO LEARN MORE

Male Cancer Survivor and Having Families: https://www.cancer.gov/about-cancer/treatment/side-effects/fertility-men

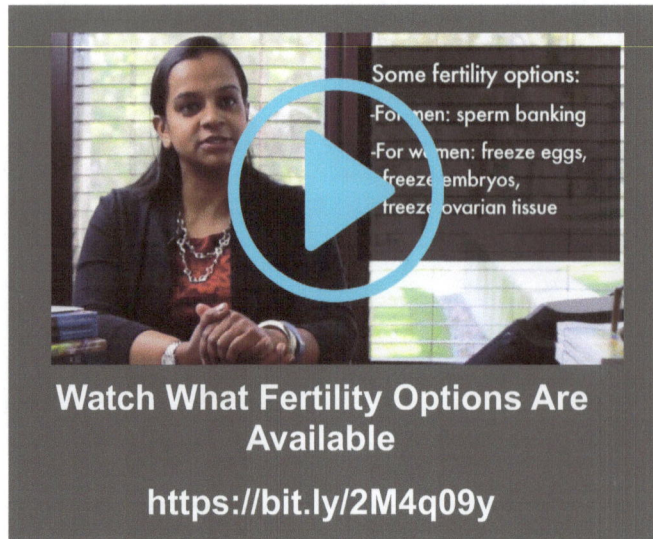

Watch What Fertility Options Are Available

https://bit.ly/2M4q09y

Making An Appointment With Your Doctor To Discuss Oncofertility

"The goals of our program are to assess every patient's risk of fertility loss, and to intervene early to integrate options into their treatment."

— Julie Messina, PA-C

Now is the time to make an appointment with your primary care physician or oncologist to discuss your options regarding fertility preservation, if you haven't already done so. Before this meeting, make sure you've done your research, and read up on the various specialists who are experts in the field of oncofertility. See the links below for more research sites.

Be sure to look at The Oncofertility Consortium website at http://oncofertility.northwestern.edu/. The information and resources there are invaluable, especially in formulating questions you will want to ask your primary care doctor and/or oncologist.

"When I got the cancer diagnosis, and found out the treatment might affect my ability to have children, my world literally stopped. I didn't know what to do, where to go or anything. I think most of us go into panic mode. The reason I say this is because after the diagnosis, we need to gather our thoughts, then make informed decisions about our future reproductive issues based on viable information."

— 28-Year-Old With Sarcoma

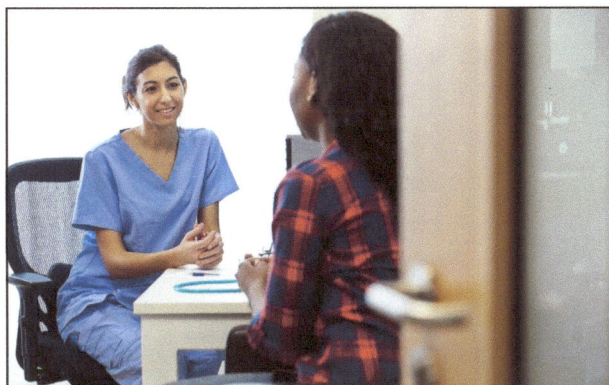

If you are a parent or a caregiver of a child who will be undergoing cancer treatment, and you have concerns about their future fertility, these instructions apply to you, too. It's possible your child will want to be part of this conversation with their doctor. They also might want to have a say, not only in their cancer treatment, but their fertility preservation. Be prepared for this.

The conversation with your primary care doctor and/or oncologist should begin by asking about their familiarity with the concept of oncofertility and fertility preservation. They should be able to recommend an oncofertility specialist. If they don't have a recommendation - or if there is no local fertility specialist who can help - The Oncofertility Consortium can guide you to an expert.

That oncofertility expert will walk you through what comes next.

Having A Conversation With Your Oncofertility Specialist

"Meaningful survivorship starts on day one. As a health care provider, I promise I will think about your life after cancer and the long-term effects of your treatment. The conversation about fertility might be difficult when you are first diagnosed and feeling overwhelmed, but I will be your advocate and help you navigate the road of choices. I am confident that you won't regret planning for your life after cancer. I am committed to ongoing research in the field and am excited to be at your side during your journey."
— *Julie Messina PA-C*

Julie Messina and Dr. Kondapalli both know that a conversation about reproductive issues and fertility concerns can be challenging when discussed with a newly diagnosed patient and their family. One of the ways they approach this situation is to ask if they can speak privately with the patient, so they have a personal one-on-one conversation.

TO LEARN MORE

The Oncofertility Consortium: http://oncofertility.northwestern.edu

Method for Cryopreservation and Recovery of Female Follicles: https://bit.ly/2QeahqJ

Bioengineering Primate Follicles: Immature Eggs to Live Birth: https://bit.ly/2NP45ZT

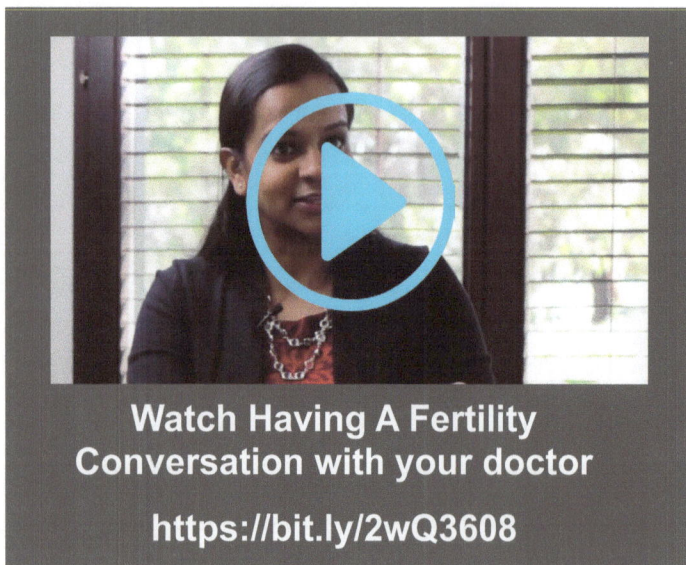

Watch Having A Fertility Conversation with your doctor

https://bit.ly/2wQ3608

If you're a young person who wants to speak freely to your doctor without your parents or caregiver present - or if you're an adult who wants some privacy with your doctor away from your family - take your doctor aside and mention it. Some doctors suggest that an individual can mention this to their doctor's receptionist when making an appointment.

After all your research, you'll want to be prepared with questions to ask your oncofertility specialist. Below are some suggestions from Dr. Kondapalli to get you started, including a few things which you should cover in the meeting. Following that is a chart with some technical medical questions regarding fertility preservation, along with an illustration on how a team of fertility specialists can work together with you and your family on specific challenges.

"The moment I met my doctor, I knew she was the one. She made me feel very comfortable. She wanted to know all about me, my family and what I was feeling about whether I wanted children in the future. Faith in your doctor is key!"

— *28-Year-Old With Lymphoma*

"Patients, especially adolescents and young adults, will often have smart questions. Not just about fertility, but safe sex practices, contraception, and reproductive health. They feel comfortable speaking privately about those issues. At the end of the private conversation, I always regroup with the family as a whole. However, patients know they have a confidential relationship with me as their provider."

— *Laxmi Kondapalli, M.D. MSCE*

"No question about your reproductive future is silly. Ask your doctors, nurses, everyone…anything you can think of!"

— *28-Year-Old With Testicular Cancer*

23

Questions for your fertility specialist:

- How is my cancer affecting my health right now?
- How quickly do I need to start treatment?
- Will my cancer or its treatment affect my future fertility?
- What fertility options are out there?
- Can I have a child after my cancer treatment?

Questions provided by MyOncofertilit.org

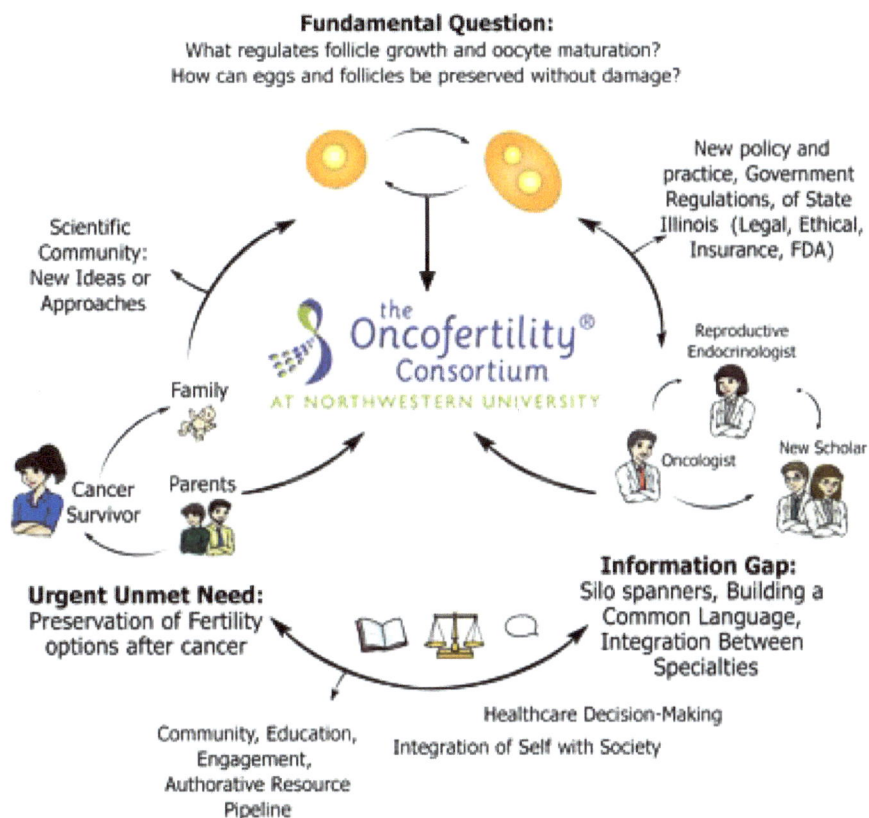

Fundamental Question:
What regulates follicle growth and oocyte maturation?
How can eggs and follicles be preserved without damage?

Scientific Community: New Ideas or Approaches

New policy and practice, Government Regulations, of State Illinois (Legal, Ethical, Insurance, FDA)

the Oncofertility® Consortium
AT NORTHWESTERN UNIVERSITY

Reproductive Endocrinologist

New Scholar

Oncologist

Family

Parents

Cancer Survivor

Information Gap:
Silo spanners, Building a Common Language, Integration Between Specialties

Urgent Unmet Need:
Preservation of Fertility options after cancer

Community, Education, Engagement, Authorative Resource Pipeline

Healthcare Decision-Making
Integration of Self with Society

TO LEARN MORE

Saving Your Fertility: https://www.savemyfertility.org/
Cancer Patients and Contraception: https://bit.ly/2xVMAw4

How Important Is It For Your Doctor To Have Oncofertility Training?

As it's probably become clear to you, the science, technology, and medicine involved in oncofertility is complicated. There are also a whole assortment of legal and ethical issues involved. Plus, there is the high cost of fertility treatments, which many insurance companies do not cover. That's why your Care Team needs oncofertility awareness.

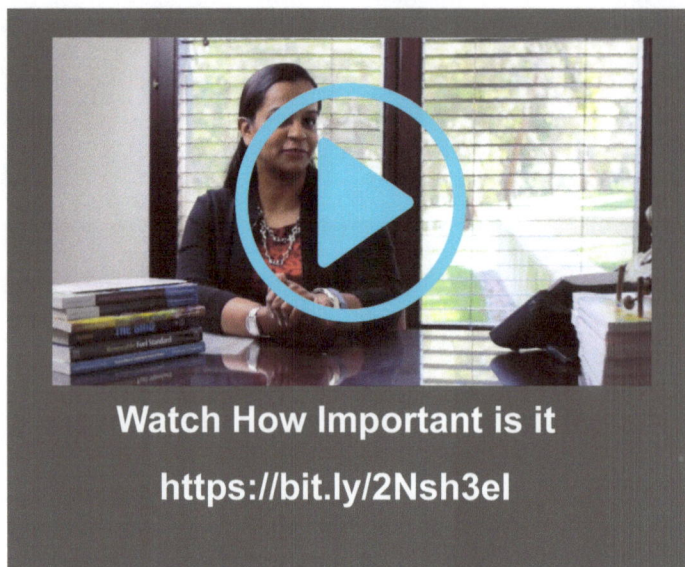

Watch How Important is it

https://bit.ly/2Nsh3el

If necessary, your team should be able to refer you to a specialist. You need someone with the right experience and the proper background in the field. You also need someone with a good understanding of the many emotional and physical consequences involved in your journey.

You also want someone who keeps current with all of the latest information and advances in oncofertility. Fertility preservation continues to quickly develop and improve, as it has in the last three to five years. Constant research in this area is active and ongoing, as we'll see below.

"I work with the cancer doctor as a part of the team that takes care of the patient. We really want families to know we are concerned about the patient's life after cancer."

— Julie Messina, PA-C

TO LEARN MORE

American Society of Reproductive Medicine: Ethic Committee Opinions: https://bit.ly/2N50QYN

AMA Journal of Ethics: Oncofertility for Adolescents: http://journalofethics.ama-assn.org/2015/09/ecas2-1509.html

How Has Fertility Technology Changed Recently?

"When I counsel patients about maximizing their future fertility potential, my first approach is to discuss and review with them the fertility preservation options that are available before they undergo their cancer treatment. In addition, I also share with them that there are many different ways of making a family - sometimes it is using your own eggs and sperm, and sometimes there are opportunities to use donor oocytes or donor sperm, or even adoption, as alternative options for parenthood."

— *Laxmi Kondapalli, M.D., MSCE*

Recently, there have been great advances in oncofertility technology. Specialists are now able to offer even more fertility preservation options for patients.

Up until 2012, oocyte cryopreservation, or what is traditionally known as egg banking, was considered experimental. But given the improvements in the way eggs are now frozen, pregnancy rates have drastically improved. The "experimental" label has since been removed from egg banking, which is now considered the standard of care.

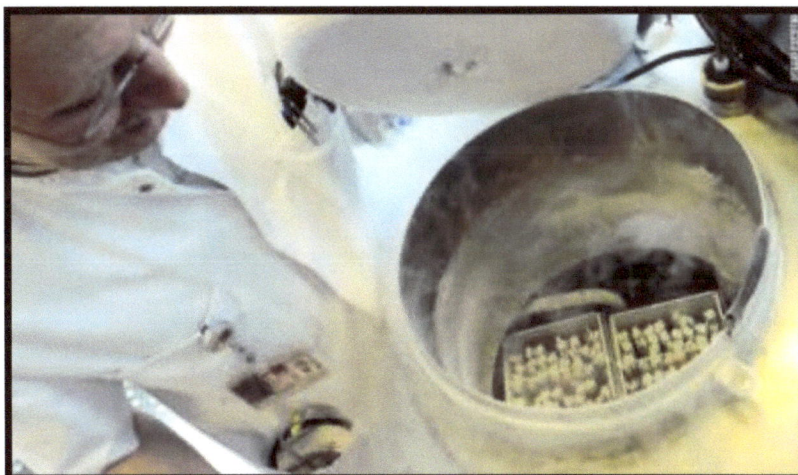

Even more encouraging, a very special first birth was recorded from transplanted ovarian tissue using ovarian tissue that was removed from a young girl before she started menstruating. Since then there have been many successful pregnancies for women using grafts of ovarian tissue.

"Depending on the type of cancer a patient has, their fertility preservation options, and the way I approach them from an oncofertility standpoint, can be quite different. For example, patients who have an abdominal or pelvic tumor may require pelvic radiation. With these patients, I would discuss a procedure called ovarian transposition. We can actually surgically suspend the ovaries to remove them outside of the radiation field."

— Laxmi Kondapalli, M.D., MSCE

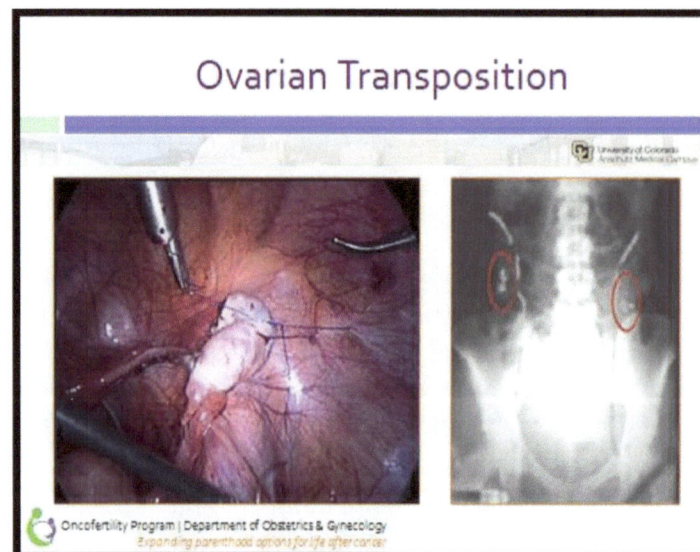

"You treat the cancer and it's over with. The fertility issue stays with you for life!"

— 32-Year-Old With Testicular Cancer

TO LEARN MORE

Egg Freezing Changing Fertility Treatments: https://www.cnn.com/2012/10/22/health/frozen-egg-banks/

Egg Freezing Puts the Biological Clock on Hold: https://n.pr/2QZWISu

Egg Freezing: A New Frontier In Fertility: https://bit.ly/2IkMjHP

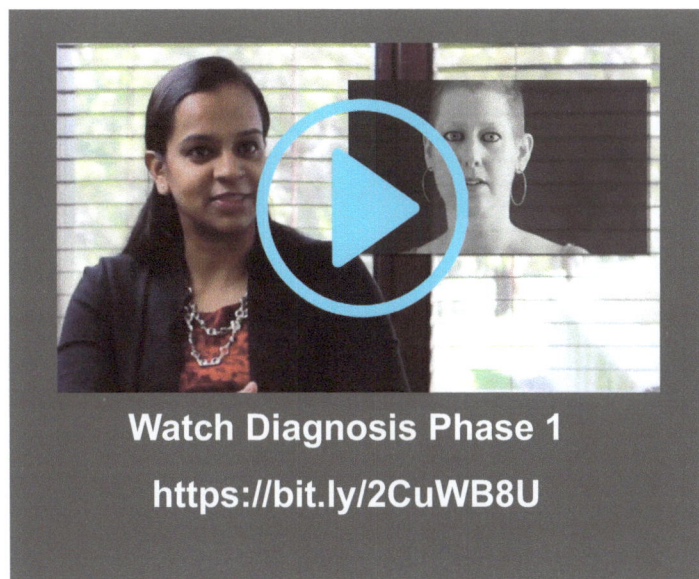

Watch Diagnosis Phase 1

https://bit.ly/2CuWB8U

Participating in the Reimagine Well Oncofertility support community gives me the opportunity to know that I'm not alone. There are other guys experiencing this in real-time. From them I can learn something, and maybe contribute to others in return."

— *29-Year-Old With Soft Tissue Sarcoma*

This is a perfect time to join Reimagine Well's Online Support Community. There are other Oncofertility patients there who've been in your shoes. They may have a lot to share with you. To create a Bridge Plan to help you get from Diagnosis to Wellbeing, go to: http://www.reimaginewellcommunity.com/reimaginewell.

Nutrition And Active Lifestyle During This Phase

"The most important things you can do to fight cancer and prepare yourself for treatment are to eat a mostly plant-based diet, maintain a healthy weight and be physically active!"

— Jocelyn Harrison, MPH, RD

Jocelyn Harrison is Reimagine Well's Nutrition, Exercise, and Lifestyle Expert. In each chapter of Part One of this book (Diagnosis, Treatment, Healing, and Wellbeing), Jocelyn will walk you through this part of your journey. Here, in the diagnosis phase, Jocelyn advises you to pick a few of the following on which to focus. Then discuss and confirm your plan with your doctor.

- Strive for a balanced diet to keep your body healthy and strong. Use Choose My Plate at https://www.choosemyplate.gov/ to plan meals that include these food groups:
    - A) Vegetables and fruit are half of your plate
    - B) Lean protein such as chicken, fish, or beans
    - C) Whole grains
    - D) Dairy/dairy alternatives w/calcium
    - E) Small amounts of healthy fats like olive oil, nuts, and avocados
- Make half your plate colorful vegetables, which are chock full of vitamins, minerals, fiber, and phytochemicals. Phytochemicals are found naturally in plants, and are powerful cancer fighters that give plant foods their color.
- Switch out sugar sweetened beverages like sodas, sports drinks, and coffee drinks for milk or water.
- Have fruit for dessert.
- If you have an exercise routine, continue it. If you don't have an exercise routine, start walking. Studies show many people with cancer feel better physically and emotionally when they get some amount of exercise each day.
- Get your information from reliable sources. Be aware of online nutrition advice or advice from well-meaning family and friends. Healthcare professionals will provide you with the most up-to-date evidence-based guidance.
- Ask your doctor if there are any diet or exercise restrictions before treatment.
- Start with small changes and don't be shy about asking for help and advice.

"A Registered Dietitian (RD) is a nutrition expert. They will have the medical expertise and time to help you devise a nutrition plan that is both satisfying and provides your body what it needs to fight cancer."

— Jocelyn Harrison, MPH, RD

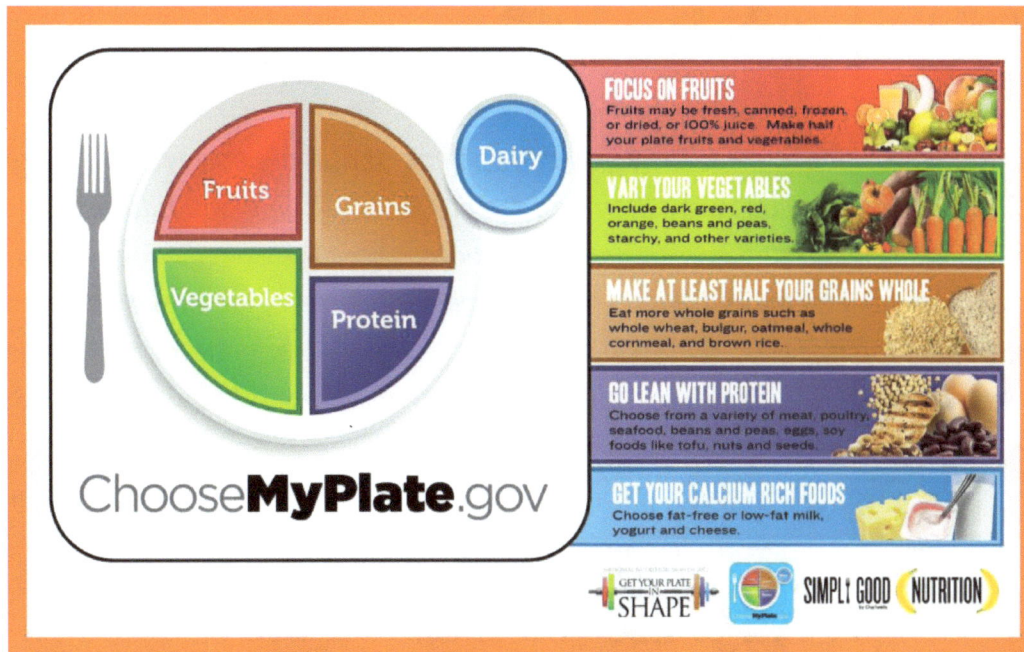

FOCUS ON FRUITS
Fruits may be fresh, canned, frozen, or dried, or 100% juice. Make half your plate fruits and vegetables.

VARY YOUR VEGETABLES
Include dark green, red, orange, beans and peas, starchy, and other varieties.

MAKE AT LEAST HALF YOUR GRAINS WHOLE
Eat more whole grains such as whole wheat, bulgur, oatmeal, whole cornmeal, and brown rice.

GO LEAN WITH PROTEIN
Choose from a variety of meat, poultry, seafood, beans and peas, eggs, soy foods like tofu, nuts and seeds.

GET YOUR CALCIUM RICH FOODS
Choose fat-free or low-fat milk, yogurt and cheese.

ChooseMyPlate.gov

GET YOUR PLATE IN SHAPE   SIMPLt GOOD NUTRITION

Here are more tips Jocelyn recommends for lifestyle changes to consider:

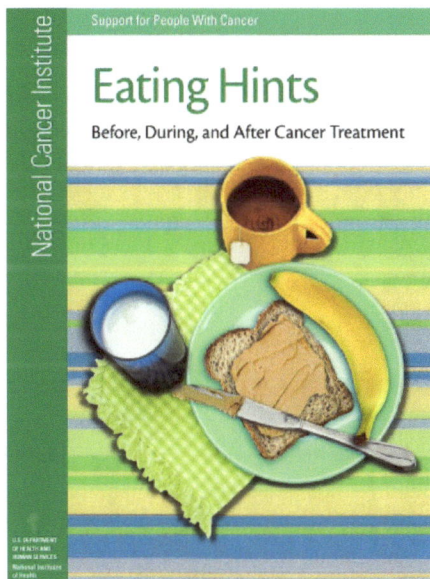

- Take on what you can. Eating a mostly plant-based diet of vegetables and fresh fruit, daily physical activity and good sleep are the foundation of fighting cancer.

- Limit the amount of processed foods like candy, cookies, pastries, sugar-sweetened beverages, and sugary coffee drinks that you consume. These foods are high in calories but low in nutrition.

- Absolutely stop smoking if you can. Cigarette smoking damages every organ in your body and is the number one cause of death you can control. Your body will have an easier time fighting cancer without the toxic effects of cigarette smoke.

- Alcohol is also toxic to your body. If you do drink, then follow the recommendation - no more than one drink for women and two for men a day.

TO LEARN MORE

Choose My Plate: https://www.choosemyplate.gov/

Cigarette smoking: https://www.cdc.gov/chronicdisease/resources/publications/aag/pdf/2016/tobacco-aag.pdf

Some Final Words of Advice

"The kinds of goals I would ask my patients to think about, especially in the diagnosis phase, are: One - consider what their desires are for children in the future; two - seek as much information and ask as many questions about the specific impact of their particular cancer treatment on long-term fertility; and, three - to make time to talk with friends, family, loved ones, or partners who are their support network, and to communally come to a decision about fertility preservation and how to proceed with fertility preservation."

— *Laxmi Kondapalli, M.D., MSCE*

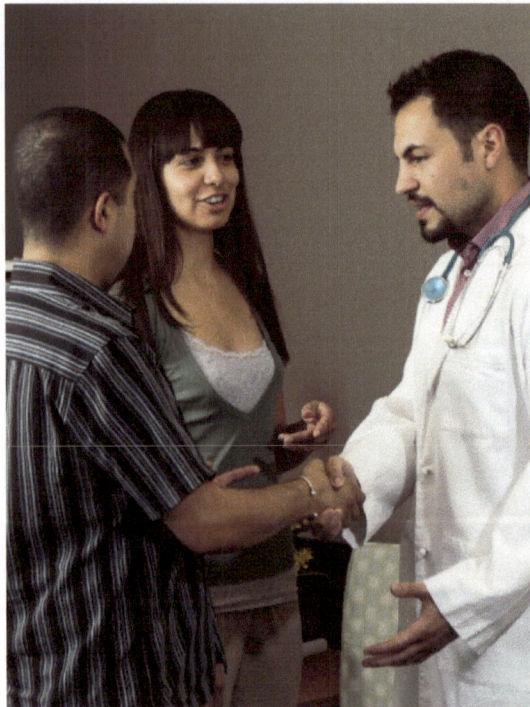

"Patients with cancer understand family is important. I think about this when each one is diagnosed and plan for their life after cancer. My heart breaks for them as we sit together and they cry because they made it through the toughest battle of their life and now, they cannot have children. Many of them have known they want to be a mom or a dad their whole lives. My goal for them is to have all the opportunities to have a family that every person, cancer or not, should have."

— *Julie Messina, PA-C*

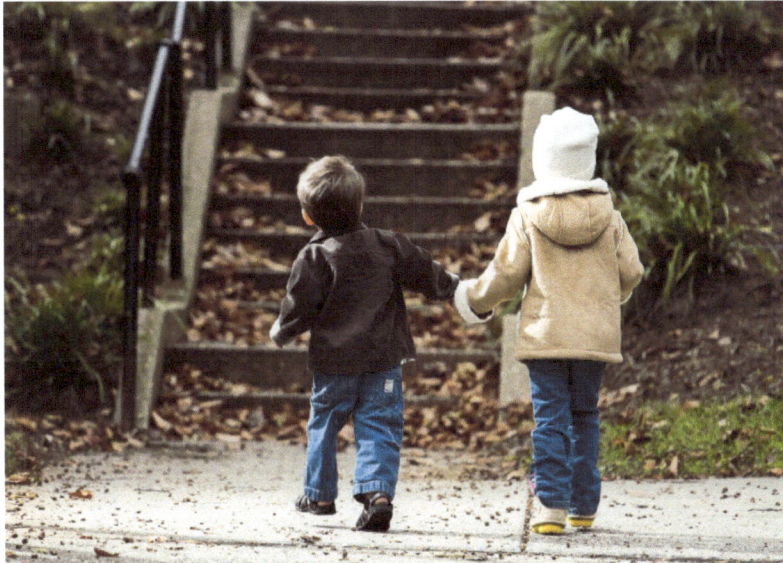

Health Goals For The Diagnosis Phase

- Think about what my plans are for children and a family in the future

- Do research about Oncofertility

- Make sure my oncologist is aware of fertility issues

- Ask questions about the impact of my type of cancer on my long term fertility

- Discuss fertility issues with my support network, partner, family, friends, and others who have been through this experience

- Make sure I take care of my new dietary, nutritional, and lifestyle changes

These are suggested goals only. Please collaborate with your support community to develop your own goals for this phase.

If you are ready to create your Bridge Plan, to help you get from Diagnosis to Wellbeing, go to: http://www.reimaginewellcommunity.com/reimaginewell

Notes

Treatment

"The way that I approach patients who are currently in treatment and desire fertility preservation is not thinking about the cancer subtype itself, but about what treatment they're receiving."

— *Laxmi Kondapalli, M.D., MSCE*

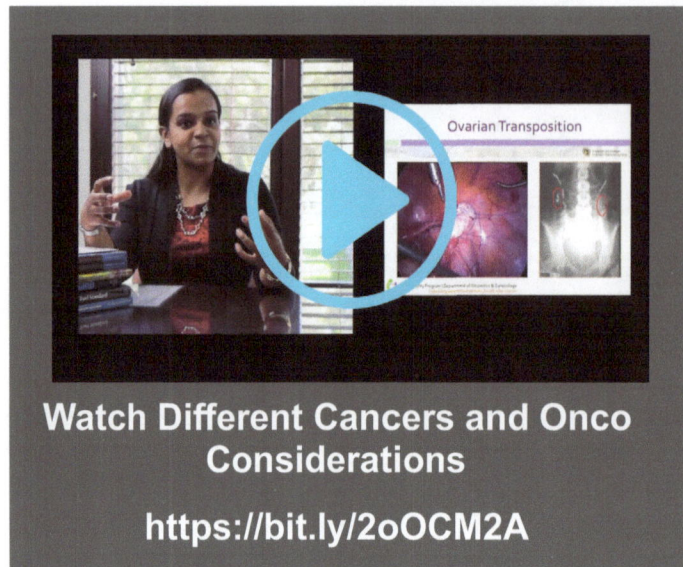

Watch Different Cancers and Onco Considerations

https://bit.ly/2oOCM2A

If you haven't done so already, the beginning of the treatment phase would be a great time to create and start working on your Reimagine Well Online Bridge Plan. Remember, the Bridge Plan is for Oncofertility cancer patients and caregivers alike. Once you join our support community, you can interact with, learn about, and get support from other cancer patients and caregivers. They've been in the exact same place you are right now!

To join up, go to: http://www.reimaginewellcommunity.com/reimaginewell

Before Cancer Treatment Begins

During the treatment phase, consideration of oncofertility issues can be quite difficult. So the best opportunity for patients to optimize their fertility preservation choices is to pursue some sort of egg, embryo or sperm banking prior to starting chemotherapy or radiation.

In other words, if you are going to freeze your eggs or sperm, or participate in any of the other medical procedures to insure that you will have a chance to have children after your cancer surgery, TALK TO YOUR DOCTOR AND DO IT BEFORE TREATMENT BEGINS. You should also let your doctor know if there may be cultural or other impediments to fertility preservation.

"Sometimes there are cultural or religious barriers. We always try to take into consideration that religion and culture will play into a patient's decision as to whether they will participate in fertility preservation. For example, some religious groups place childbearing at the highest level of importance. Others may forbid masturbation, which is necessary for sperm collection. We make an effort to be sensitive to patients in all of these situations."

— Julie Messina, PA-C

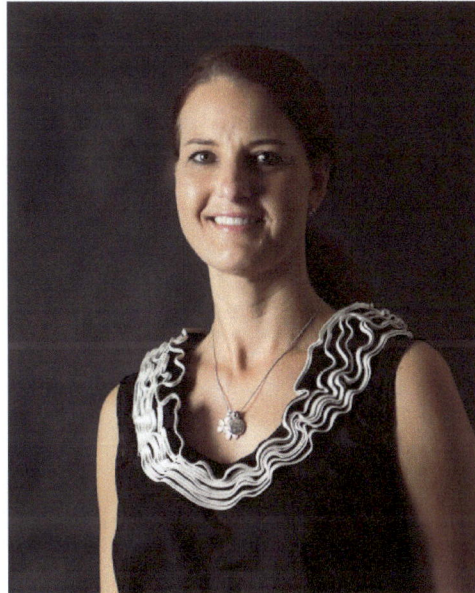

Oncofertility Concerns During Treatment

If you are still considering your options, or wish to try oncofertility procedures during or after your therapy, these are some of the concerns of which to be aware:

- During cancer treatment, most of the egg and sperm banking choices (or the new procedures with ovarian and testicular tissue freezing) that can be offered are not as successful or appropriate as the same procedures done before cancer treatment begins.
- Young women who wish to undergo egg banking during treatment may not be able to do that. Some of the hormonal medications needed to stimulate the eggs in a woman's ovaries to grow will not work during cancer treatments.
- Even if the ovaries can produce mature eggs, the quality of the eggs may be questionable. These eggs will have been exposed to radiation or chemotherapy, thereby causing unknown changes to the DNA in the eggs.
- Young men who wish to do sperm banking during cancer treatment often find there is no sperm in their specimen samples to freeze.
- Even if a young man can produce sperm during cancer treatment, that sperm will have been exposed to radiation and chemotherapy. The quality of the sperm will be unknown.

"For a patient who has a hematologic cancer such as leukemia or lymphoma, the options that I discuss with them might be a little bit different. For example, ovarian tissue freezing is an option that is available for leukemia or lymphoma patients, even in a pediatric population. However, the successful pregnancies that have occurred from using frozen tissue have resulted from transplantation. Unfortunately, patients who have blood-borne malignancies really aren't candidates for transplantation. The last thing that we would want is for a patient to overcome their cancer and then potentially re-introduce those malignant cells through the transplanted tissue."

— Laxmi Kondapalli, M.D., MSCE

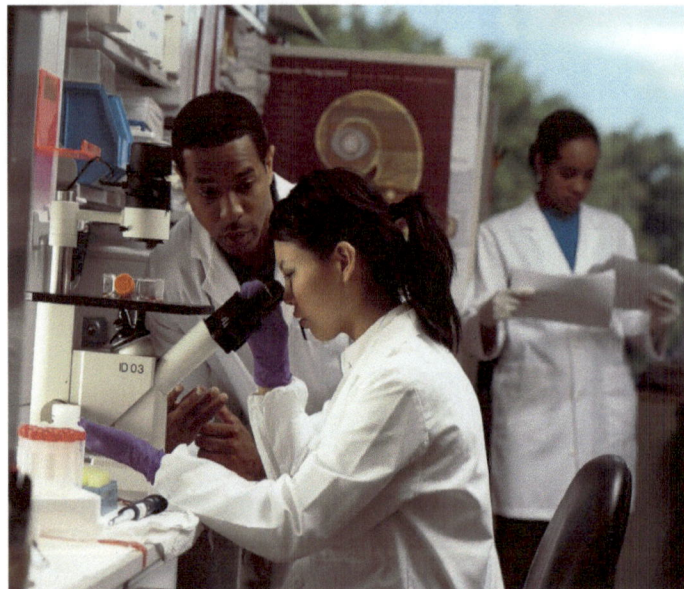

"One example of potential damage done to a woman's fertility during cancer treatment would be a patient who receives cyclophosphamide, an alkylating chemotherapeutic agent that is widely used in a variety of different cancers. Cyclophosphamide can have an impact on the eggs that remain within the ovary. So, regardless of the type of cancer a patient has, a woman who has been exposed to cyclophosphamide may not respond to fertility treatment."

— Laxmi Kondapalli, M.D. MSCE

TO LEARN MORE

More information on Cyclophosphamide and its Effects: https://medlineplus.gov/druginfo/meds/a682080.html

Male Fertility and Cancer Treatment: https://www.oncolink.org/support/sexuality-fertility/fertility/male-fertility-and-cancer-treatment

Take Care Physically, Mentally and Emotionally

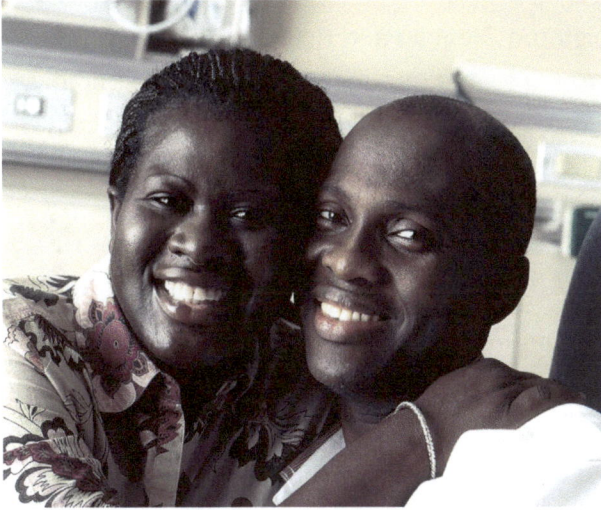

Because of the stressful concerns you may have before and during the treatment phase of your cancer journey, the Reimagine Well Team recommends that you take care of yourself physically, mentally, and emotionally. That means eating well to keep up your strength, staying as active as possible, surrounding yourself with people who are supportive and helpful, and making arrangements to see a mental health expert. Be aware that it's going to take everything you've got to get through your cancer treatment. Do not be afraid or feel any shame about talking to a therapist, psychologist, social worker, or anyone on your Care Team. That also applies to talking about your oncofertility and reproductive health issues.

"We talk about other sexual health with our adolescent, young adult, and adult patients. Preventing pregnancy during therapy, as well as sexually transmitted diseases, are discussed. Our team also discusses how to maintain intimate relationships during a patient's treatment."

— Julie Messina, PA-C

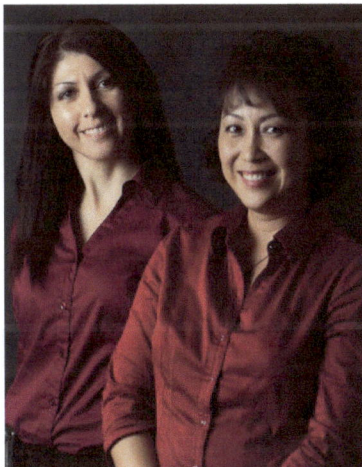

This would also be a great time to create a Reimagine Well Online Bridge Plan at https://www.reimaginewellcommunity.com/reimaginewell. There are cancer patients there just like you, who know and understand what you're going through. This includes issues regarding Fertility Preservation.

TO LEARN MORE
Counseling Services You May Need: https://bit.ly/2OTTjhb
Emotional Side Effects: https://bit.ly/2DCtgdg

Nutrition And Active Lifestyle During This Phase

Jocelyn Harrison, Reimagine Well's resident Registered Dietitian and Active Lifestyle Expert, shares a lot of information that will be helpful as you enter the treatment phase. It is extremely important that during this time you take the best care of yourself that you can, both physically and emotionally.

"Plan to have a conversation with your doctor about what to expect during treatment in terms of your diet and nutrition; also about your physical activity."

— *Jocelyn Harrison, MPH, RD*

Here's a list of questions to ask your doctor before treatment begins:

- Are there any changes I should make to my current diet?
- Should I be taking a multivitamin? (If you are taking supplements of any kind, bring a list of what you are taking and share it with your health practitioner and dietitian.)
- If my treatment is causing me to vomit often, should I be concerned about getting enough nutrients?
- Should I try liquid meal replacements if I have trouble keeping solid food down?
- What if I just don't feel like eating much for a couple days after treatment?

During treatment, you often have to eat foods that are different than what is considered "healthy". You will need to eat to keep your strength up and deal with the side effects of treatment. You might have a problem eating enough food, so you may need extra protein and calories. Treatment with chemotherapy and radiation is designed to kill cancer cells, but it can also harm healthy cells. Damage to healthy cells can cause side effects that may lead to eating problems. Here are some types of eating problems that cancer treatment may cause:

- Appetite loss
- Change in sense of taste or smell
- Constipation
- Diarrhea
- Dry Mouth
- Fatigue
- Feeling full quickly
- Food aversions
- Lactose intolerance
- Nausea
- Sore mouth, tongue, or throat
- Trouble swallowing
- Vomiting
- Weight gain
- Weight loss

Always talk to your doctor, nurse or dietitian about any problems on this list. There are specific steps to address each of these side effects. A dietitian can help you make changes to your diet to minimize the nutritional impact of side effects. Be wary of online nutrition advice or advice from well-meaning family and friends. Healthcare professionals will provide you with the most up-to-date evidence-based guidance.

"Studies show many people with cancer feel better when they get some exercise each day. Talk to your Care Team about an exercise plan that is right for you."

— Jocelyn Harrison, MPH, RD

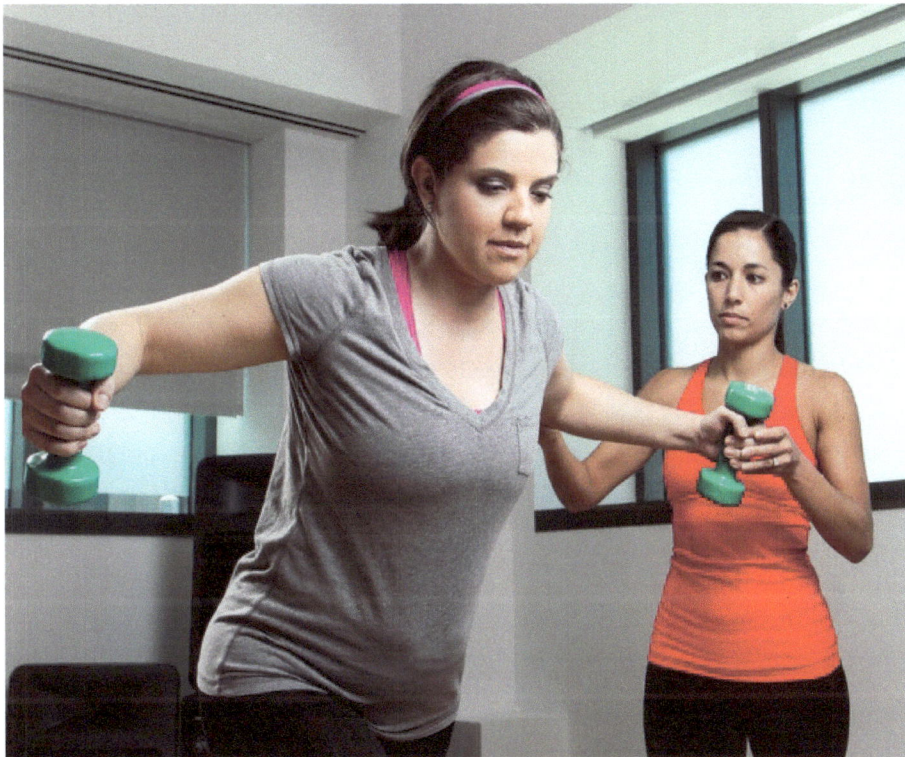

Once you've had that discussion about your exercise plan, put it into motion.

- Write out your exercise plan.
- Keep a journal about your daily progress.
- Use an online fitness app like My Fitness Pal to keep track of your physical activity and diet.
- Use a paper calendar and write down your goals or activities for the day.
- Use a fitness tracker or pedometer that tracks your steps.
- Use your Reimagine Well Online Support Community to form a group and help each other achieve realistic health goals during treatment.

Complementary and Alternative Medicines (CAMs)

You may be wondering whether you should consider using alternative medical therapies that you have read about, are interested in trying, or may already be practicing. These can include massage, relaxation exercises, vitamins, acupuncture, and homeopathic medications. They are officially referred to as "complementary" and "alternative" medicines (CAMs).

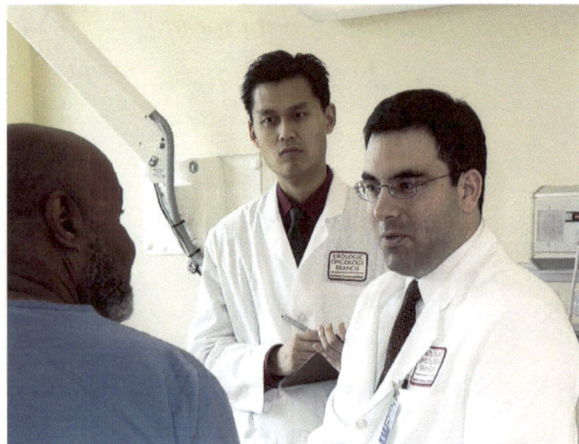

Before including any CAMs in your treatment you should always discuss them with your doctor and Care Team. Give your doctor, nurse or dietitian a list of vitamins, minerals, dietary supplements, herbs or alternative therapies you are doing, or are interested in doing.

Some CAM approaches, such as therapeutic massage, have been proven to be safe and effective. Stick to the therapies that have been researched. A good place to start your personal research on this is the National Cancer Institute's CAM page.

There are no studies, however, that prove that using any special diet, food, vitamin, mineral, dietary supplement, herb, or combination of these can slow cancer, cure it, or keep it from coming back. As a matter of fact, some of these products can cause other problems by changing how your cancer treatment works. Your doctor can help you avoid dangerous drug-drug or drug-food interactions. If you're using a CAM now, let your doctor know.

"Many dietary supplements contain levels of antioxidants (such as vitamins C and E) that are much higher than the recommended Dietary Reference Intakes for optimal health. There is a concern that antioxidants might repair the damage to cancer cells that cancer treatments cause, making the treatments less effective. However, at this time the science is unclear, so it is best to avoid supplements that provide more than 100% of the Daily Value for antioxidants."

— Jocelyn Harrison, MPH, RD

TO LEARN MORE

Nutrition in Cancer: https://www.cancer.gov/about-cancer/treatment/side-effects/appetite-loss/nutrition-pdq#section/_125

Dealing With Treatment Side Effects: https://bit.ly/2Oh9S9D

My Fitness Pal: https://www.myfitnesspal.com

Complementary and Alternative Medicines (CAMs):https://www.cancer.gov/publications/dictionaries/cancer-terms?CdrID=44384

National Cancer Institute's CAM page: https://www.cancer.gov/about-cancer/treatment/cam

Dietary Reference Intakes: https://www.cancer.gov/publications/dictionaries/cancer-terms/def/dietary-reference-intakes

Reimagine Well Online Support Community: http://www.reimaginewellcommunity.com/reimaginewell.

Future Oncofertility Treatments

"There are promising future fertility preservation options that are coming down the pike. We are now able to isolate individual eggs from the outer layer of the ovary. There are opportunities to actually grow those immature eggs completely in an in vitro or lab system. That is a technology that has advanced over the last three to five years. Great advancements are continuing to happen in this area. On the male side, there are new technologies to actually biopsy or remove portions of the testes in prepubertal young males. That tissue can be frozen, and then transplanted back into the testes, where mature human sperm can be created. These options are still experimental, but I believe over the next few years these options are going to be a reality."

— Laxmi Kondapalli, M.D., MSCE

"I am confident that someday in the future, scientists will discover how to reverse infertility!"

— 20-Year-Old With Anaplastic Large Cell Lymphoma

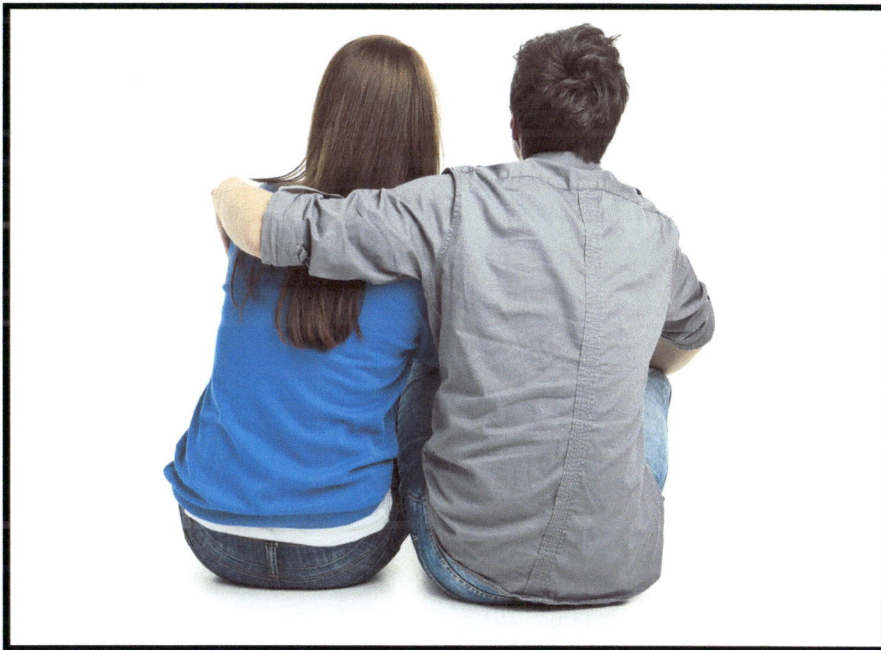

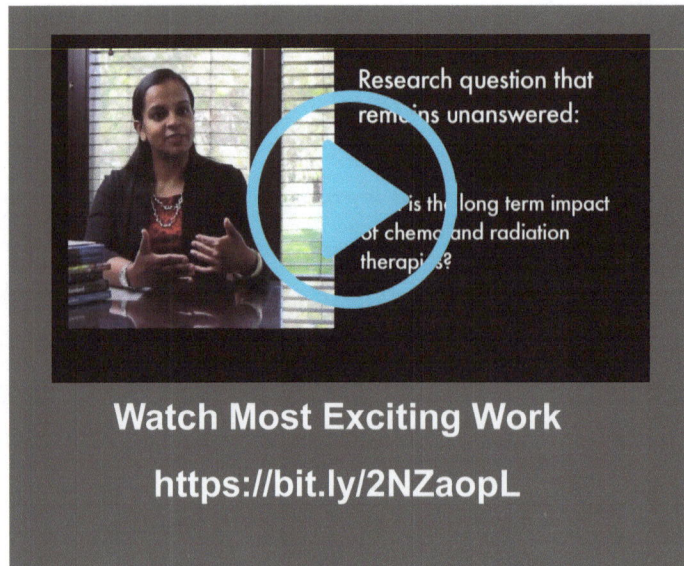

Watch Most Exciting Work

https://bit.ly/2NZaopL

Health Goals For The Treatment Phase

- Plan my fertility preservation procedures like egg and sperm banking before treatment begins
- Take care of my physical health by eating well and exercising, as per my doctor's recommendations
- Take care of my mental health by talking to an oncofertility specialist, an oncology social worker, psychologist or therapist
- Take care of my social health by joining a support group or a social group for people who understand what I've been through

These are suggested goals only. Please collaborate with your support community to develop your own goals for this phase.

If you want to create your Bridge Plan now, to help you get from Diagnosis to Wellbeing, go to: http://www.reimaginewellcommunity.com/reimaginewell

Notes

Notes

Healing

"After completing their therapy, a cancer patient or a survivor - from a reproductive standpoint - still may be facing the long-term side effects from their treatment."

— *Laxmi Kondapalli, M.D., MSCE*

Before moving into the Healing Phase, if you would like to join Reimagine Well's Online Support Community and create a Bridge Plan to get you from Diagnosis to Wellbeing, go to: http://www.reimaginewellcommunity.com/reimaginewell

What About Side Effects After Treatment?

During the healing phase, side effects from your cancer treatment, particularly those affecting fertility issues, can impact your quality of life. These side effects may continue for some time. You might exhibit high levels of anxiety and stress, plus issues with physical and emotional pain, fatigue, and sexual problems.

"For many of my female patients, they may stop getting their period during chemotherapy or radiation. Their periods may not come back for 6 to 12 months after cancer therapy. During the time when their periods have not started again, they might not feel like a normal person. So they may have unnecessary concern or anxiety about the fact their body hasn't gotten back to normal."

— *Laxmi Kondapalli, M.D., MSCE*

These side effects can affect you if you are a male, too. If you are having sexual problems, discuss them with your primary care doctor, oncologist, or even seek out an oncofertility specialist, if you already haven't. A psychologist can also help address these challenges.

"We must address sexual health after cancer treatment. Many male patients experience sexual dysfunction and low libido. We work with psychologists and urologists to help address these issues."

— *Julie Messina, PA-C*

TO LEARN MORE
Perception Of Fertility Affects Quality Of Life In Young, Female Cancer Survivors: https://bit.ly/2xHqJct
Life After Cancer Treatment And Ways To Manage Physical Changes: https://bit.ly/2pH0758

Family Planning Conversations

"Patients come see me after they've completed their therapy so we can regroup. I discuss contraceptive options, particularly since many oncologists advise patients to postpone pregnancy for one to two years after completion of their therapy. That can be a challenging conversation to have. Some of the options may not be appropriate for particular cancer patients. Patients who have had different types of chemotherapy may not be appropriate candidates for certain types of contraceptive methods."

— *Laxmi Kondapalli, M.D., MSCE*

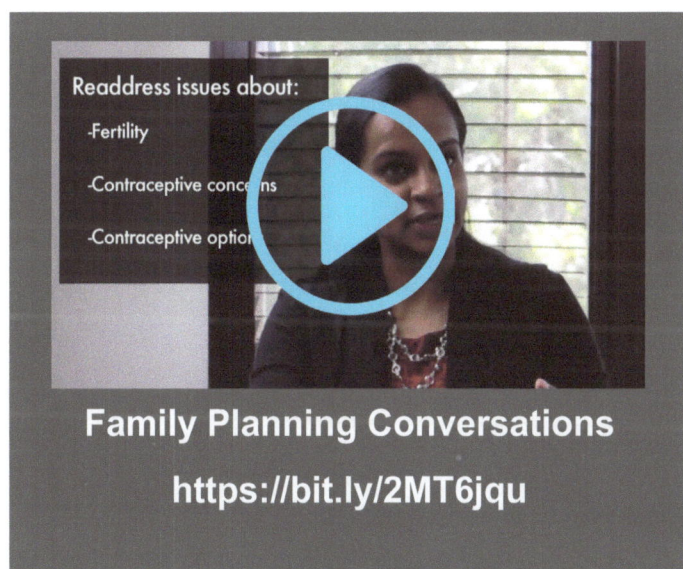

Readdress issues about:

-Fertility

-Contraceptive concerns

-Contraceptive options

Family Planning Conversations
https://bit.ly/2MT6jqu

As Dr. Kondapalli notes, you may be advised to put off your plans to have a child for up to two years after your treatment ends. This may happen because of chemotherapy, radiation, or other treatments you've had.

Putting off having a child means having a conversation with your doctor about family planning. Family planning usually means the use of contraception (in any of its various forms) to avoid a pregnancy. Sometimes there are cultural or religious barriers to practicing contraception. Or there may even be medical barriers, such as interactions between particular medications.

When you have this conversation with your doctor, oncologist, or anyone on your Care Team, if your religion or culture has objections to contraception in any form, you need to let them know.

The conversation may indeed be challenging, but you and your Care Team must work together on this. Don't be afraid or embarrassed to talk about any issues involving family planning.

48

Get Counseling About Pregnancy

So you've waited the 12 to 24 months after finishing your treatment, as recommended. Maybe you've started to think about your future. Perhaps you are about to begin another round of tests to see how your fertility levels are doing. Maybe you already had the tests, and are about to start a family. You might be scared, nervous, excited, apprehensive, or all of those things.

Wherever you are in your oncofertility journey, it's also important to take into consideration the type of treatment you received - whether it was a low, intermediate, or high risk for infertility.

Now is the time to discuss all the possible options and outcomes of a pregnancy with your doctor and your Care Team, before you make the next move. It's crucial to get this counselling so you can make a smart, thoughtful decision about your future. Information is your best friend.

"I refer my female cancer survivors to a specialist, who has expertise in the safety of pregnancy after cancer, known as a Maternal Fetal Medicine provider, for preconception counseling."

— *Laxmi Kondapalli, M.D., MSCE*

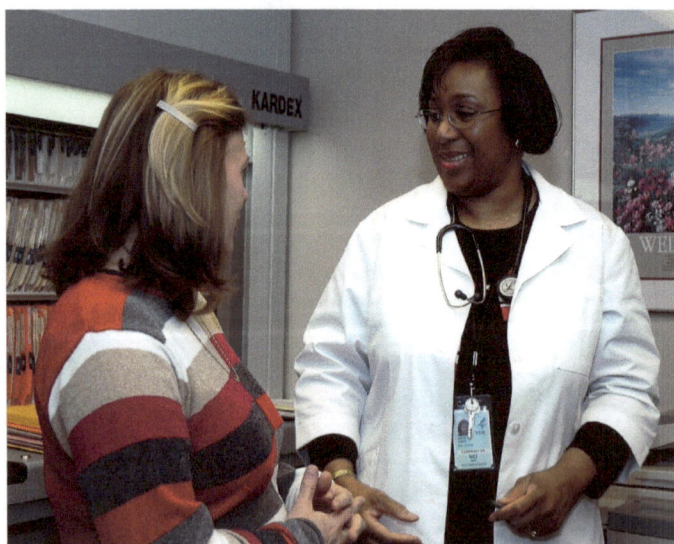

TO LEARN MORE
Having A Baby After Cancer: http://www.cancer.net/survivorship/life-after-cancer/having-baby-after-cancer-pregnancy
Managing Pregnancy After A Cancer Diagnosis: https://bit.ly/2NJTKOP

What If A Survivor Hasn't Had Fertility Preservation?

"It's important to understand some female survivors may have a very small window of fertility because of the damage done from chemotherapy to the eggs in their ovaries."

— Julie Messina, PA-C

If you're in the healing phase and haven't had a conversation with your oncologist about fertility preservation, start that conversation right away. There still may be options that you and your doctor can discuss. A good place to begin is a talk about your fertility status. Once that is known, then other options can be considered.

"There are a number of things I can provide, like blood tests and ultrasounds, for my female patients. For my male patients, something as simple as a semen analysis to assess their current status. This can be done in their cancer healing phase."

— Laxmi Kondapalli, M.D., MSCE

"When I found out later that I needed to freeze my embryos, my initial reaction was to be upset that we didn't take action ahead of time."

— 32-Year-Old With Hodgkins Lymphoma

TO LEARN MORE

What Young Cancer Patients Aren't Being Told About Their Fertility: https://cbsn.ws/2ImV6sT

Female Fertility Preservation: https://www.livestrong.org/we-can-help/just-diagnosed/female-fertility-preservation

Nutrition and Active Lifestyle During This Phase

"As a result of your cancer treatment you may have lost or gained weight beyond what is healthy. One important part of cancer prevention or preventing a recurrence is to maintain a healthy weight."

— Jocelyn Harrison, MPH, RD

After treatment, your body needs to recover. It may be some time before it's 100% of what it was. A good goal for your healing phase is to safely return to your optimal health. To get you back to that, there are many different diets and active lifestyle choices. No one size fits all. So Reimagine Well's nutrition and lifestyle expert Jocelyn Harrison has suggestions on how to get you back on the road to wellbeing.

Goals to Reduce Future Cancer Risk

Jocelyn recommends these goals from the American Institute for Cancer Research (AICR):

- Be as lean as possible without becoming underweight.
- Be physically active at least 30 minutes a day. Moderate-intensity cardiovascular activity five times a week; muscle-strengthening exercises two days a week.
- Eat a large variety of vegetables, fruits, whole grains, and legumes/beans.
- Avoid sugary drinks.
- Limit consumption of energy-dense or salty foods, particularly processed foods high in added salt, sugar, fat, and low in fiber.
- Limit consumption of red meats and avoid processed meats.
- Limit alcoholic drinks.
- Do not rely on supplements to protect you against cancer.
- Do not smoke or chew tobacco.

"Be patient with yourself and your progress. Remember, changing behavior takes time. By making gradual changes you are much more likely to stay on track in the long run."

— Jocelyn Harrison, MPH, RD

TO LEARN MORE

American Institute for Cancer Research: http://www.aicr.org/reduce-your-cancer-risk/recommendations-for-cancer-prevention/
Recommendations for cancer prevention: http://www.aicr.org/reduce-your-cancer-risk/recommendations-for-cancer-prevention/

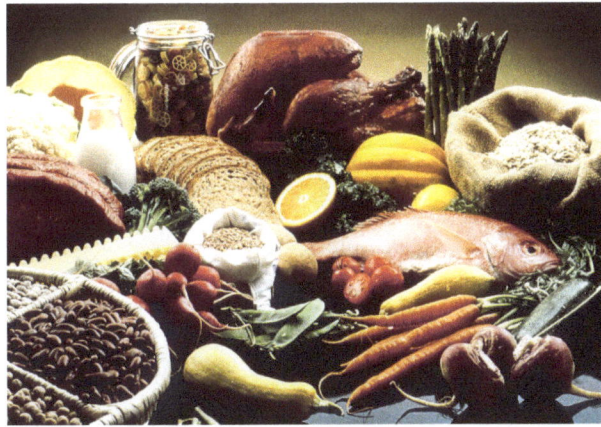

Most Important Dietary Goals

You don't have to become a vegetarian or give up the foods you love, says Jocelyn. It's your overall pattern of eating that counts.

- Vegetables, fruits, whole grains, and beans should always take up at least 2/3 of your plate. To maximize vitamins and minerals, choose colorful produce such as dark leafy greens, tomatoes, strawberries, blueberries, carrots, and cantaloupe.
- Fish, poultry, lean red meat, cheese, and other animal foods should take up only 1/4 or less of your plate. Try to go meatless several times a week.
- Prepare your own food. The best way to know what's in your food is to make it yourself. There are endless ways to create fresh wholesome meals.

"Depending on the type and location of your cancer, your may have had surgery that alters your digestive system. For example, stomach cancer may require that part of the stomach be removed. Be sure to ask your doctor if your treatment impacts the way you can eat. Ask for a referral to a Registered Dietitian (RD) to get a healthy eating plan based on the specifics of your treatment regimen."

— *Jocelyn Harrison, MPH, RD*

Most Important Physical Activity Goals

You don't have to join a gym or buy equipment to exercise. Physical activity can be low-cost or free. An old pair of supportive rubber-soled shoes and an exercise DVD or Youtube video can start you on your way. Any sidewalk can be an Olympic track.

- Break up your 30 minutes of daily activity into 10-to-15 minute sessions. This provides the same health benefits. If you sit a lot, take walks every two hours.
- Use physical activity as your personal "me" time. Or you may get more motivated by joining a class or having an activity buddy. Either way… exercise!
- If you resolve to exercise for 30 minutes a day and then miss a day, don't give up. Forgive yourself and get back to it! Try a different time of day if that works for you.

Specific Goals Are The Best Goals!

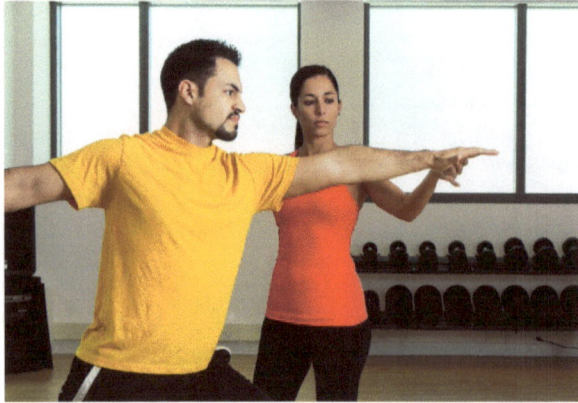

- Focus on individual goals. Don't try to make huge, drastic changes overnight.
- Ask for help. Find a registered dietitian (RD) and a certified exercise physiologist.
- Go public with your health goals. If you have joined the Reimagine Well Support Community, there is a place on your Bridge Plan to document your goals and share them with friends and family.
- Tell others about your goals and let them help you achieve them.
- Record your behavior. Track your progress or change your goal if you need to.
- Reward yourself when you reach milestones along the way to your goal.
- Accept setbacks, work through them, then get back on track!

"My recommendation is to find others who can relate to your fertility issues - whether it be online or in person. Read about other people's reproductive stories. Talk with loved ones. Never stop trying and believing."

— *20-Year-Old With Anaplastic Large Cell Lymphoma*

Health Goals For The Healing Phase
- Think about what my family goals are for the future
- Seek out my fertility options
- Meet with my doctor or provider about family planning and contraception options
- Take care of my physical, dietary and sexual wellbeing
- If I didn't take care of fertility preservation before treatment, look into other options during healing

These are suggested goals only. Please collaborate with your support community to develop your own goals for this phase.

If you are ready to create your Bridge Plan, to help you get from Diagnosis to Wellbeing, go to: http://www.reimaginewellcommunity.com/reimaginewell

Notes

Notes

Wellbeing

"In the wellbeing stage, I would advise female patients to follow up with their obstetrician. For some, I recommend seeking the advice and consultation of a maternal fetal medicine doctor. They specialize in high-risk obstetrics… about how patients who have a whole host of medical illnesses might still have a safe pregnancy."

— Laxmi Kondapalli, M.D., MSCE

You've probably already joined the Reimagine Well Online Support Community. If you haven't, you're missing out on something that many people like you on the oncofertility cancer journey have found to be helpful. Other cancer patients and survivors are there, along with caregivers, asking and answering questions, posting blogs and Tips 4 Life. Maybe you're a private person, or maybe you just haven't had the time to create your Bridge Plan. Find the time.

Go to: http://www.reimaginewellcommunity.com/reimaginewell

Current Fertility Status

"I advise male and female patients to first identify their current fertility status. Get information from primary care physicians or fertility specialists. Find out and assess what the long-term impact cancer treatment may have had on your fertility."

— Laxmi Kondapalli, M.D., MSCE

Most oncologists and fertility specialists recommend that once you have finished your treatment, you wait a while before you consider your pregnancy options. Often that is because side effects can last a while, and can affect your fertility.

"When I found out the chemo had rendered me infertile, it was very upsetting. It was definitely hard to take at first. I was confused and angry. I kept asking "Why me?"

— 20-Year-Old With Anaplastic Large Cell Lymphoma

"If the initial evaluation shows decreased fertility, ongoing assessments can occur. This can continue up to a five-year period post-treatment. It can take take that long before the effects are better understood."

— Julie Messina, PA-C

Pregnancy Consideration

If you have already pursued fertility preservation prior to your cancer treatment, the wellbeing phase may be an opportunity for you to actually use some of your banked eggs, embryos, or sperm. Now's the time to have a talk with your primary care doctor or oncofertility specialist.

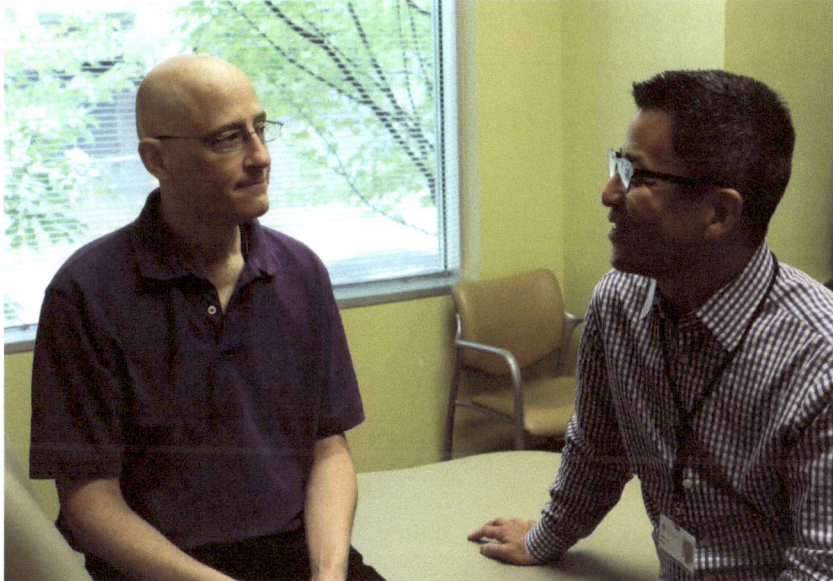

Some Cancer Subtypes That May Affect Your Fertility

"Some of my young Hodgkin's/lymphoma patients have been exposed to certain types of chemotherapy that can have toxic effects either on their lungs or even on their heart. During pregnancy, the blood volume is increased by fifty percent because so much of that blood volume and nutrients are there to support the growing pregnancy."
— *Laxmi Kondapalli, M.D., MSCE*

Whether you are waiting for some time to pass before you can get a fertility assessment, or have already been cleared by your doctor and Care Team to start trying to get pregnant, there may be some additional hurdles to your ongoing pregnancy considerations. One hurdle may be that some cancer subtypes can interfere with fertility treatment.

TO LEARN MORE

Pregnancy After Cancer: https://www.nccn.org/patients/resources/life_after_cancer/pregnancy.aspx

Your Fertility: http://www.myoncofertility.org/articles/if_my_male_partner_has_been_treated_cancer_does_mean_he_infertile/

"For my young patients who have been exposed to Adriamycin, there are baseline tests we can do to assess their cardiac function even before considering pregnancy. We can be sure to monitor them and be aware of any complications they may be at risk for during pregnancy. For patients who have had pelvic radiation, one thing I discuss with them is that radiation exposure can predispose them to certain pregnancy complications, such as preterm birth or having a small baby. Patients need to be aware of these things on their fertility journey."

— Laxmi Kondapalli, M.D., MSCE

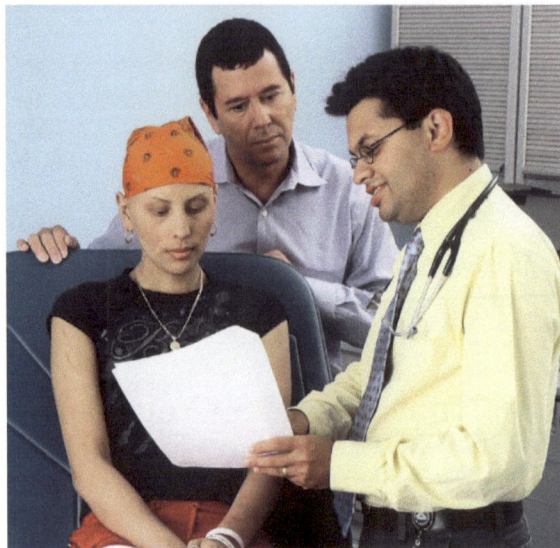

Talk to your doctor for more information about these conditions, and any other concerns you might have regarding fertility.

"New studies are looking at some long-term side effects, not only on fertility and reproductive function, but on hormonal production, and how that may predispose young patients to early diabetes or heart disease, as well as the impact on bone health. Researchers think from a fertility standpoint about how the area of hormonal production can impact other important body systems."

— Laxmi Kondapalli, M.D., MSCE

Finding Your "New Normal"

Here at Reimagine Well, we use a term called "The New Normal." Your new normal will define what you are capable of now that your cancer therapy has ended, you have moved from your healing into your wellbeing phase, and you are looking forward to your Survivorship. This is the time to learn how to maximize your potential to live a healthy, normal life.

You'll find your new normal by learning what you are capable of doing, mentally, physically, and emotionally. Go slow in the beginning. Take your time. See what you're feeling. Then begin to push yourself a little more every day. Finding your new normal doesn't happen instantly. It's a process where you get in touch with your new body and your new life.

You will also find a new normal when dealing with fertility concerns, particularly in regard to issues such as contraception, when and how to start a pregnancy, temporary or permanent infertility and what to do when discussions about adoption or surrogacy need to take place.

"My chemotherapy-induced infertility is something it took me a while to comprehend and live with. But I've learned to accept it and find an alternative way to build a family!"
— 27-Year-Old With Anaplastic Large Cell Lymphoma

What finding your new normal really means is moving into your future. As you do this, be sure you follow your survivorship treatment plan, go to your medical appointments, and make sure your doctor looks for any long-term side effects that may appear years after your treatment.

Most importantly, remember that no matter what happens, as you move into the future there are many oncofertility paths available to you. Stay positive, seek out all the experts you can, and know, as Dr. Kondapalli reminds us, that you are not alone!

"For cancer survivors in the wellbeing phase, they may have trouble resuming their normal lives because they've undergone a tremendously difficult experience. Doctors like myself are here to help them. I would advise patients to maintain certain health goals. One is a healthy lifestyle: eating well, exercising, and making sure that they are able to enjoy doing their normal activities. Two, I would advise patients to find out their fertility status if pregnancy and future fertility are of concern to them. And three would be to seek out information from doctors and reliable medical sources. Then they can discuss next steps with their primary care physician. They can also seek the expertise of a fertility specialist. I would also advise patients to join oncofertility support groups or get involved in their local oncofertility community! "

— *Laxmi Kondapalli, M.D., MSCE*

"With the technology that exists today, incredible new fertility treatments and options are becoming available every day!"

— *20-Year-Old With Anaplastic Large Cell Lymphoma*

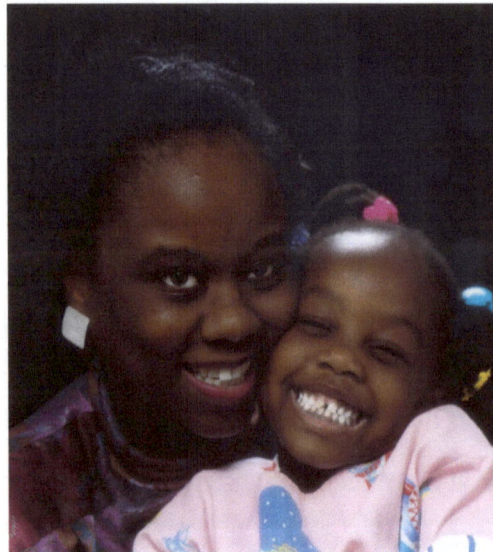

TO LEARN MORE

Young Cancer Patients and Survivors Take Part in Oncofertility Research: https://bit.ly/2R4XmlU

Oncofertility Consortium and Research: http://oncofertility.northwestern.edu/for-researchers

Mentoring Others

Mentoring is a process by which you share your own medical experiences with another patient or caregiver. By mentoring them, you empower them. The same way you were empowered. You give them hope. And you strengthen them for what lies ahead.

You can mentor others by volunteering at the hospital where you or your loved one was treated, or at your own local hospital or medical center. You can help in an online community or by phone.

Giving back not only helps another person, it helps you as well.

"There are phenomenal peer-to-peer programs where they can also shepherd another young person who's newly diagnosed and has been through or will go through many of the same experiences that they have. It's a great opportunity for those young people to provide that same type of support to future patients."

— *Laxmi Kondapalli, M.D., MSCE*

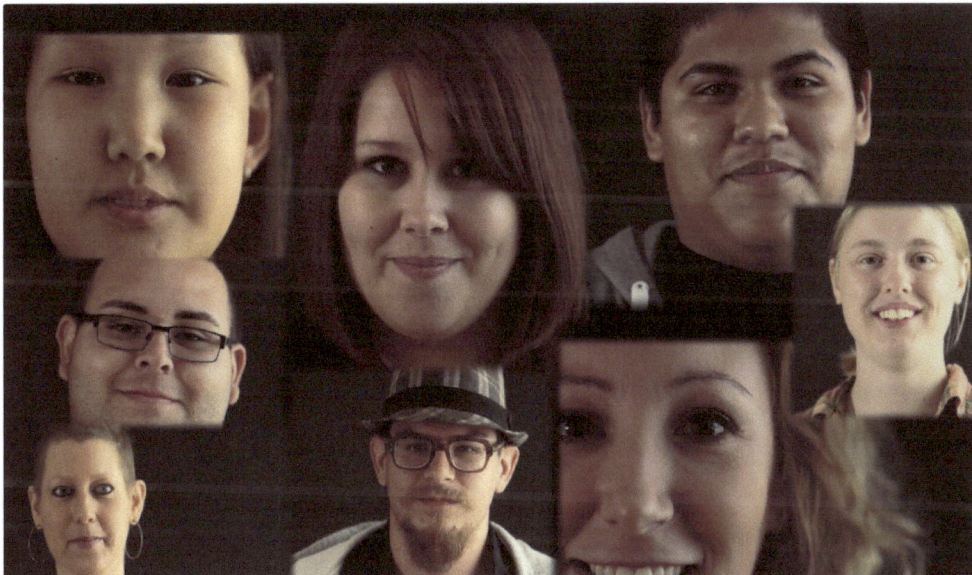

TO LEARN MORE

Adolescents and Young Adults With Cancer: https://www.cancer.gov/types/aya

4th Angel – Patient & Caregiver Mentoring Program: http://www.4thangel.org/

Cancer Connects Volunteer Mentor Program: http://www.cancerconnects.org/volunteerMentorProgram

Imerman Angels: http://imermanangels.org/

Nutrition/Active Lifestyle - Link To Previous Material

In the wellbeing phase, it is time to solidify a healthy diet and exercise plan that supports your health but also fits into your life for the long run. Focusing on healthy lifestyle habits is your key to preventing a cancer recurrence.

A healthy diet and a physically active life is even more important if children are a part of your future. Current science tells us that the health of both the mother and father before conception has a big impact on the long-term health of their children.

You can incorporate healthy habits that you have developed over your cancer journey. We suggest that you revisit the Nutrition and Active Lifestyle section in the previous chapter of this Learn Guide.

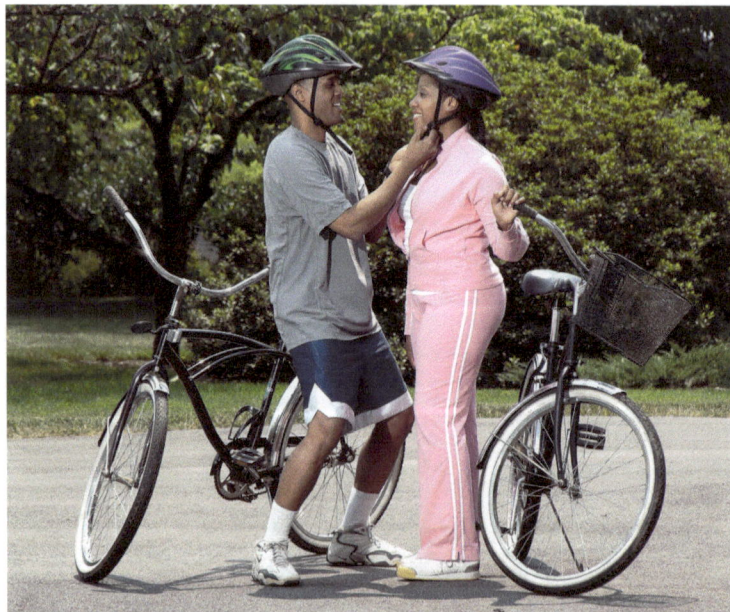

Our Online Support Community

As you finish this part of the Learn Guide, we again would like to suggest you visit our Reimagine Well Support Community. It's where patients, survivors, caregivers, and healthcare professionals share their knowledge. To reach the support community, go to http://www. reimaginewellcommunity.com/reimaginewell

Watch Health Goals During the Wellbeing Phase...

https://bit.ly/2QcBaMw

Health Goals For The Wellbeing Phase

- Develop a healthy diet
- Develop and maintain a proper exercise program
- Enjoy my normal activities
- Check my fertility resources
- Keep on eye out for long-term side effects from my treatment
- Follow up with my survivorship plan
- Go to my survivorship medical appointments
- Consider mentoring cancer patients following in my footsteps
- Consider participation in post-treatment studies
- Join support groups and get involved in my community

These are suggested goals only. Please collaborate with your support community to develop your own goals for this phase.

Closing Words From Our Oncofertility Specialists

"The most important thing to communicate to a newly diagnosed patient is that they have options available to them. These are choices we can work on together to make really informed decisions about their reproductive health in the future. There are experts and professionals available to help them and shepherd them through a very difficult process."

— Laxmi Kondapalli, M.D., MSCE

"I love my patients. Patients with cancer have been sent down a path they didn't choose. Somehow they seem to find the strength within to fight for life. My patients teach me so much about love, family, friendship, determination, appreciation, and myself."

— Julie Messina, PA-C

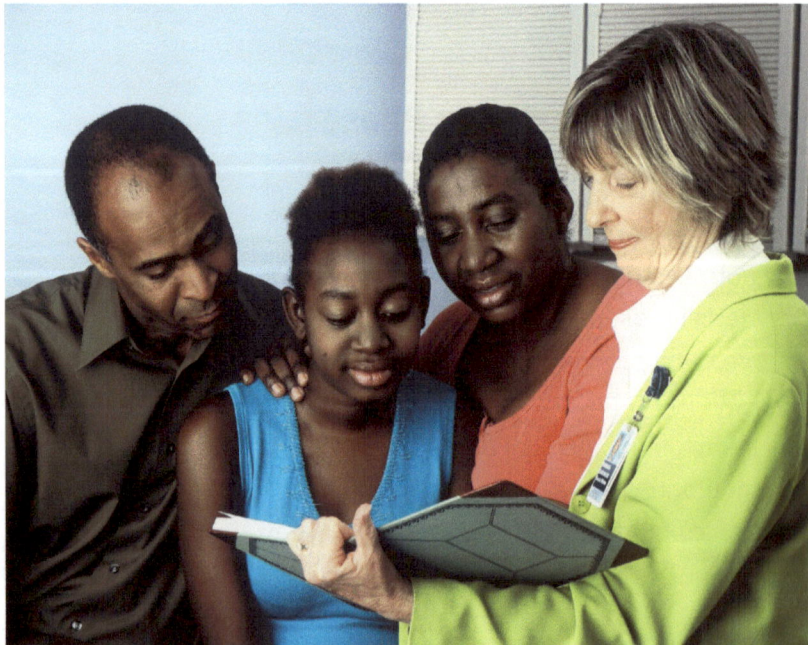

Here's the Science

We know there are those of you, whether patients, caregivers, or family members, who want to dig a little deeper into the details of oncofertility. There are also individuals who are interested in the pure science of this new, emerging medical field.

Below, Reimagine Well's expert Julie Messina shares information with you that goes beyond what was discussed earlier in the Learn Guide. It's evidence-based scientific reading for anyone who would like to learn a little more. You'll find footnotes included.

PRIMARY OVARIAN INSUFFICIENCY

In a recent medical review, it was reported that the North American Children's Oncology Group considers the risk of primary ovarian insufficiency to be highest with busulfan administered at a dose of at least 600 mg per square meter of body-surface area, cyclophosphamide at a dose of at least 7.5 g per square meter, or ifosfamide at a dose of at least 60 g per square meter, but an international multidisciplinary panel reached no consensus on this matter. (1)

Pelvic radiotherapy is also known to cause premature ovarian insufficiency, since exposure to 5 to 10 Gy is toxic to oocytes. Indeed, the human oocyte is very sensitive to radiation — a dose of less than 2 Gy is estimated to be sufficient to destroy 50% of primordial follicles. (2,3)

OVARIAN RESERVE AND PRIMARY OVARIAN INSUFFICIENCY

Ovarian reserve refers to the population of primordial follicles - which have the potential to develop into an egg - present in a human female. A female fetus has the highest number of follicles - approximately seven million - about five months before she is born. This count slowly drops so that at a female's birth, 85% of these follicles have been lost.

The average age of menopause for women in America is 51. We now know that it isn't age that determines when menopause begins, but the number of follicles a woman has remaining inside her. Researchers have determined that approximate follicle number to be about 1000. This information is relevant because the probability that primary ovarian insufficiency will develop after cancer treatment is related to the ovarian reserve. (4)

References

1. van Dorp W, Mulder RL, Kremer LCN, et al. Recommendations for premature ovarian insufficiency surveillance for female survivors of childhood, adolescent, and young adult cancer: a report from the International Late Effects of Childhood Cancer Guideline Harmonization Group in collaboration with the PanCareSurFup Consortium. J Clinical Oncology 2016;34:3440- 50.

2. Wallace WH, Thomson AB, Kelsey TW. The radiosensitivity of the human oocyte. Human Reproduction 2003;18:117-21.

3. Donnez J, Dolmans MM. Preservation of fertility in females with haematological malignancy. Br J Haematol 2011;154: 175-84.

4. This is from a talk Julie Messina and our other oncofertility expert Laxmi Kondapalli attended a few years ago. Further information is from Wallace WH, Kelsey TW. Human Ovarian Reserve From Conception To The Menopause. PLoS One 2010;5(1):e8772.

UPDATED CONSENSUS ON THE RISK OF PREMATURE OVARIAN FAILURE

The current, updated consensus from the North American Children's Oncology Group regarding which medications and procedures pose the highest risk of premature ovarian failure are as follows: Busulfan, administered at 600 mg/metered squared of body surface area; Cytoxan, 7.5 gram per meter squared; and Ifosfamide, at a dose of 60 grams per meter squared. Pelvic radiation at 5-10 Gy is toxic to oocytes. (5)

GONADOTOXICITY IS AGE DEPENDENT

First line treatment does not compromise ovarian reserve by more than 10% in girls under age 10, whereas girls who are 11 or 12 have an estimate 30% on decline of their ovarian reserve. (7,8, 9)

WHICH STRATEGY OF EGG FREEZING AND THAWING IS ACCEPTED AS BEST?

Oocyte vitrification and warming is superior to slow freezing and thawing in terms of clinical outcomes. (6)

References

5. van Dorp W, Mulder RL, Kremer LCN, et al. Recommendations For Premature Ovarian Insufficiency Surveillance For Female Survivors Of Childhood, Adolescent, and Young Adult Cancer: A Report From The International Late Effects of Childhood Cancer Guideline Harmonization Group in collaboration with the PanCareSurFup Consortium. J Clinical Oncology 2016;34:3440- 50.

6. Rienzi L, Gracia C, Maggiulli R, et al. Oocyte, Embryo and Blastocyst Cryopreservation in ART: Systematic Review And Meta-analysis Comparing Slow-Freezing Versus Vitrification To Produce Evidence For The Development Of Global Guidance. Human Reproductive Update 2017;23:139-55.

7. Wallace WH, Kelsey TW, Anderson RA. Fertility Preservation In Pre-Pubertal Girls With Cancer: The Role Of Ovarian Tissue Cryopreservation. Fertility And Sterility 2016; 105:6-12.

8. Wallace WH, Smith AG, Kelsey TW, Edgar AE, Anderson RA. Fertility Preservation For Girls And Young Women With Cancer: population-based validation of criteria for ovarian tissue cryopreservation. Fertility and Sterility 2016

9. El Issaoui M, Giorgione V, Mamsen LS, et al. Effect of first line cancer treatment on the ovarian reserve and follicular density in girls under the age of 18 years. Fertility And Sterility 2016; 106(7):1757-1762.e1.

Notes

Notes

"If you or somebody you care about has been diagnosed with cancer, we're here to help you get from diagnosis to wellbeing."

— Team Reimagine Well

In Part One of this Learn Guide, our goal was to supply you with informational and educational material regarding how to deal with your Oncofertility status, before and after your cancer treatment. We also gave you important questions about Oncofertility to ask the various doctors with whom you've been interacting. Our goal was to help you become an empowered patient or caregiver. An empowered patient or caregiver is able to actively participate in the ongoing health care decisions that have become a part of your life during your cancer journey. If you are struggling with questions about the future of your fertility, this journey can be particularly difficult. It's painful for caregivers as well, as you watch your loved ones make decisions that none of you ever thought would be a part of your family's future.

In Part Two of the Learn Guide, Reimagine Well will provide you with the steps to create a safe, private place to gather your community. You can then use their strength, wisdom, and knowledge as you move through your own, or your loved one's, cancer journey. Our patient and family support platform will also guide you in setting achievable health goals at each phase of your journey. For caregivers, you can share your experiences and feelings with other parents, guardians, and family members. You are not alone.

This step-by-step guide will help you get started on your **Reimagine Well Bridge Plan**: your health plan for life. Keep it on your phone or tablet. Print it out, phase by phase, as a chronicle of your journey to wellbeing.

All of the blogs and tips for life you'll find here have been reviewed by our medical staff and/or the National Cancer Institute prior to being published. If you need assistance at any point along the way, you can contact a member of our staff via the "Connect" link on our website at www. ReimagineWell.com.

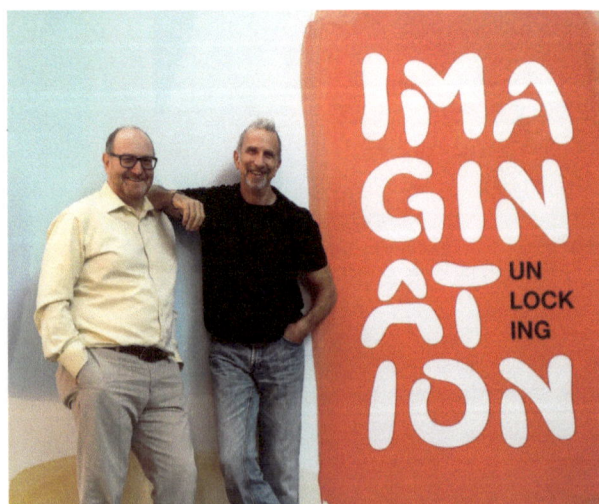

Yours In Health,
Leonard Sender, MD and Roger Holzberg -
Co-Founders

Survival UP!

Reimagine Well's support community eases the overwhelming nature of a life-threatening diagnosis by dividing the journey into manageable phases. It assists with setting achievable health goals in each phase for you, along with your caregivers, supporters, community, and healthcare professionals.

And it builds your health plan for life in the process.

Our support community also enables healthcare professionals to continue guidance post-treatment, through the healing and wellbeing phases of the journey.

We promised you at the start of this Learn Guide you would not be alone.

You're not. We're here. And so are many, many others who have been here before you.

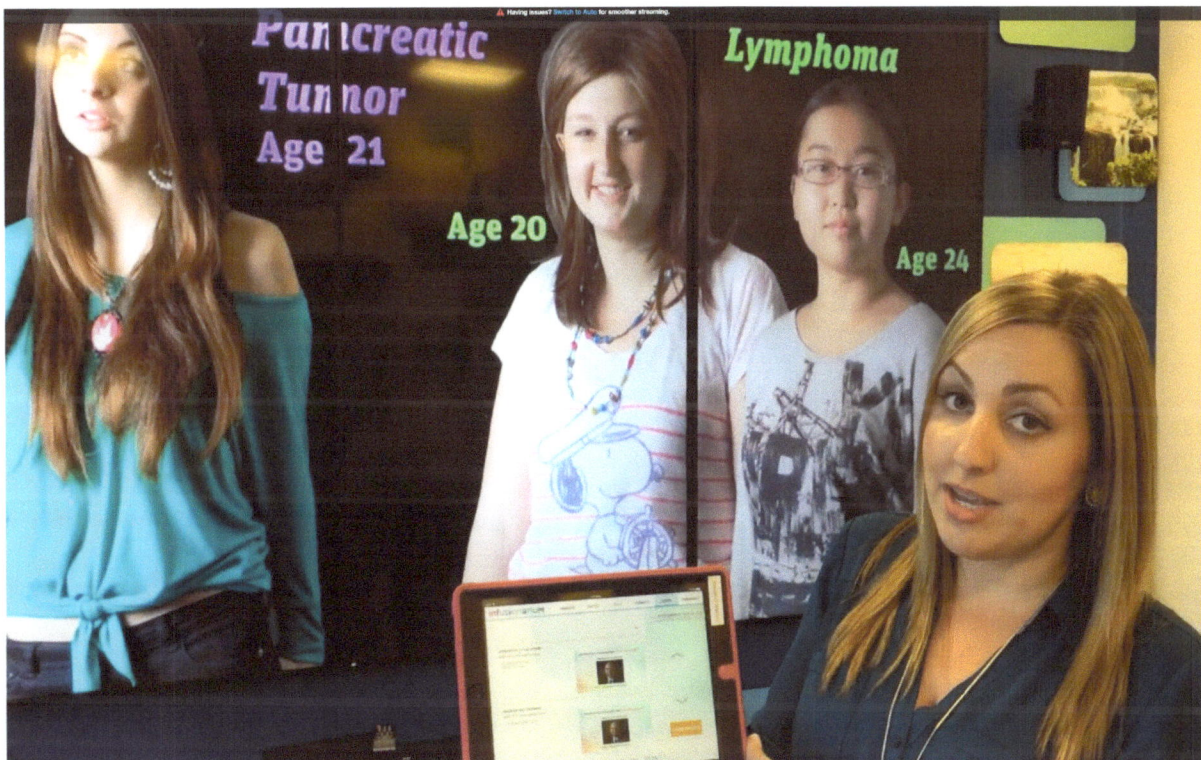

From Diagnosis to Treatment, Healing and Wellbeing

"Fertility Preservation doctors can guide patients through a difficult journey into a meaningful and joyful life!"

— Julie Messina, PA-C

"You have to become empowered to ask the right questions, and to find the right questions to get the information you need."

— Leonard Sender, M.D.

"When you're in the heat of battle… remember why you're fighting!"
— 24-Year-Old With Colon Cancer

"I knew I needed to hear what my doctors were saying, but just as important to me was what others, just like me, did to get through the minefield I was about to walk into… Empower yourself!"
— Roger Holzberg, Co-Founder and Cancer Survivor

"I gathered my family… my caregivers and my friends… and I made my plan… the most important thing is to figure out your battle plan."
— 19-Year-Old With Leukemia

"With Fertility Preservation, you have choices that weren't even available five years ago!
— Laxmi Kondapalli, M.D., MSCE

"Keep being strong and spreading the message."
— 21-Year-Old With Lymphoma

"By making gradual changes you are much more likely to stay on track in the long run."
— Jocelyn Harrison, MPH, RD

"Glad to see you on this site. Looking forward to helping each other."
— 31-Year-Old With Liver Cancer

Notes

Notes

Getting Started On Your Bridge Plan

The Reimagine Well Community™ is a private online and offline (printed book) guided support network that helps patients transition from diagnosis to wellbeing. Reimagine Well's patient and caregiver support community is a safe place for patients, families, and staff to:

- Offer support to one another
- Set achievable health goals in each phase of their cancer journey
- Share best-practices for others following in their footsteps
- Print their guide as a chronicle of the journey from diagnosis to wellbeing

"This is an amazing tool and resource for newly diagnosed patients and their families. I know that my journey would have been so much different if I'd had this support when I was just starting out."

— 37-Year-Old With Colorectal Cancer

Creating Your Bridge Plan

To become a part of the Reimagine Well Support Community go to
http://www.reimaginewellcommunity.com/reimaginewell

If you're just getting started, once you're registered, the first thing we can do is to reduce your sense of isolation by helping you build your support community.

The next few pages are the technical stuff. (All of it is contained in the Help section of the Support Platform, too.) If you have ever made a Facebook, Instagram, YouTube, Twitter, or other social media account, you'll fly right through this part!

NOTE: Unlike any other social media platform:

- Your personal data will never be shared
- You will never have sales ads "served" to you
- All Blogs & Tips 4 Life have been reviewed by healthcare professionals or the National Inst. of Health before publishing

Fill In The Personal Information

You'll be asked for the following information. Make sure it's all handy.

- Name
- Username (create a "username" if you are uncomfortable using your real name)
- Email (plus confirm email)
- Password (plus confirm password - you'll choose your own)
- Date Of Birth (you can choose to hide this)
- What Your Role Is (Patient, Caregiver, Individual, Healthcare Professional)
- Dealing With (your diagnosed illness)
- Brief Description
- Location (you can choose to hide this)
- Enter the Code (to prove you are a real person)

Reimagine Well Community
EVOLVING THE PATIENT JOURNEY

Search   Free - Get Started Now!

About Me

Name*

Type / Brief Description

About text formats

Dealing With*   I am a*
- Please Select -   - Please Select -

Date of Birth*   Location*
Hide Date of Birth   - Please Select -

Location*   Date of Birth*
Hide Location   mm/dd/yyyy

Registration Is Complete

As soon as you register and hit "Submit" you will be taken to your Bridge Plan. Yellow boxes there will include a few tips on how to start your Bridge Plan. Once you leave this page, the yellow boxes will disappear. You can get them back in "Help." And you will receive an email containing login links and more. If you don't see the email in your inbox, check your spam folder.

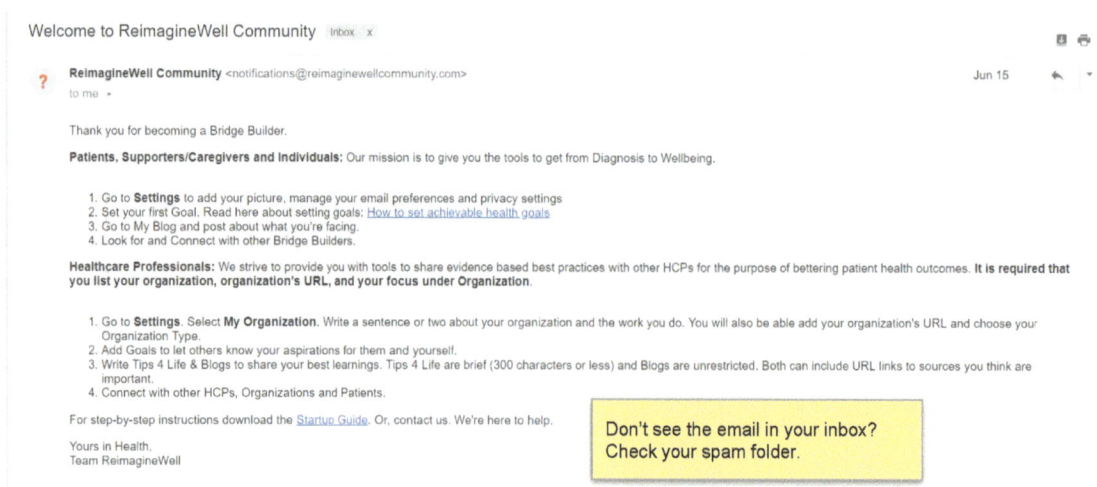

To Personalize Your Plan

To personalize your Bridge Plan, click on Settings in the top navigation box. Providing more information on your Bridge Plan will allow easier access to the people, resources, and information that are relevant to you.

Some questions will include whether you are a patient (that is anyone who has received a diagnosis), a Caregiver or Supporter (any family members or friends who support patients), Individuals (which is anyone interested in a building a Bridge Plan and using the resources of the support network), or Healthcare Professionals (who are those in the healthcare field).

There are also tabs here for Privacy Settings, which allow you to decide which information you want to receive from other Bridge Builders, and A Description Of Your Illness, where you may describe the type of illness for which you are being treated, or that of the patient you are supporting. You MUST always **Save** your changes.

> *"The Reimagine Well support network helped me pull together my team, my strongest allies, and then helped me create my battle plan."*
>
> *— 38-Year-Old With Breast Cancer*

GaryC
Patient

Edit

About Me   Password & Settings   Picture   Notification Settings

About Me

Adding personal information about yourself will enable Reimagine Well Community to better recommend other bridge builders and services to you.

I AM A: (below) enables you to choose your role. Patients are anyone who has received a diagnosis. Supporters/Caregivers include family members and friends who help support Patients. Individuals can be anyone interested in building a Bridge Plan and using the resources of Reimagine Well Community™. Healthcare Professionals are those who are in the healthcare field and would like to contribute in the community as a Healthcare Professional.

Name★

Gary

I am a★

Patient ⌄

Date of Birth★

● Hide Date of Birth
○ Show Date of Birth

Date of Birth★

07/03/2004

Location★

● Hide Location
○ Show Location

Location★

US - California ⌄

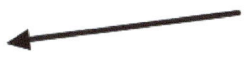

Save   **You must SAVE changes**   Cancel account

Passwords and Settings

Regarding your username. <u>If you are not comfortable using your real name, you may create a fictional username instead.</u>

Passwords. Everyone has a million of them. You should write down your Password and Username in a safe place in case you forget it. If you need to change your original password, you may do that in Settings. If you forget your password, you can request another at the bottom right of the login screen.

Your email address will be kept private and is never shared with anyone else.

If you add or change something in Settings, always hit the Submit button to save those changes. Always remember to **Save** your changes.

Picture or Photograph

You may add a picture or photo on the Settings page. A photo is a good way to personalize your Bridge Plan. As with your Username, use an "avatar" photo if you aren't comfortable with using your own image. Then **Save** the added photo.

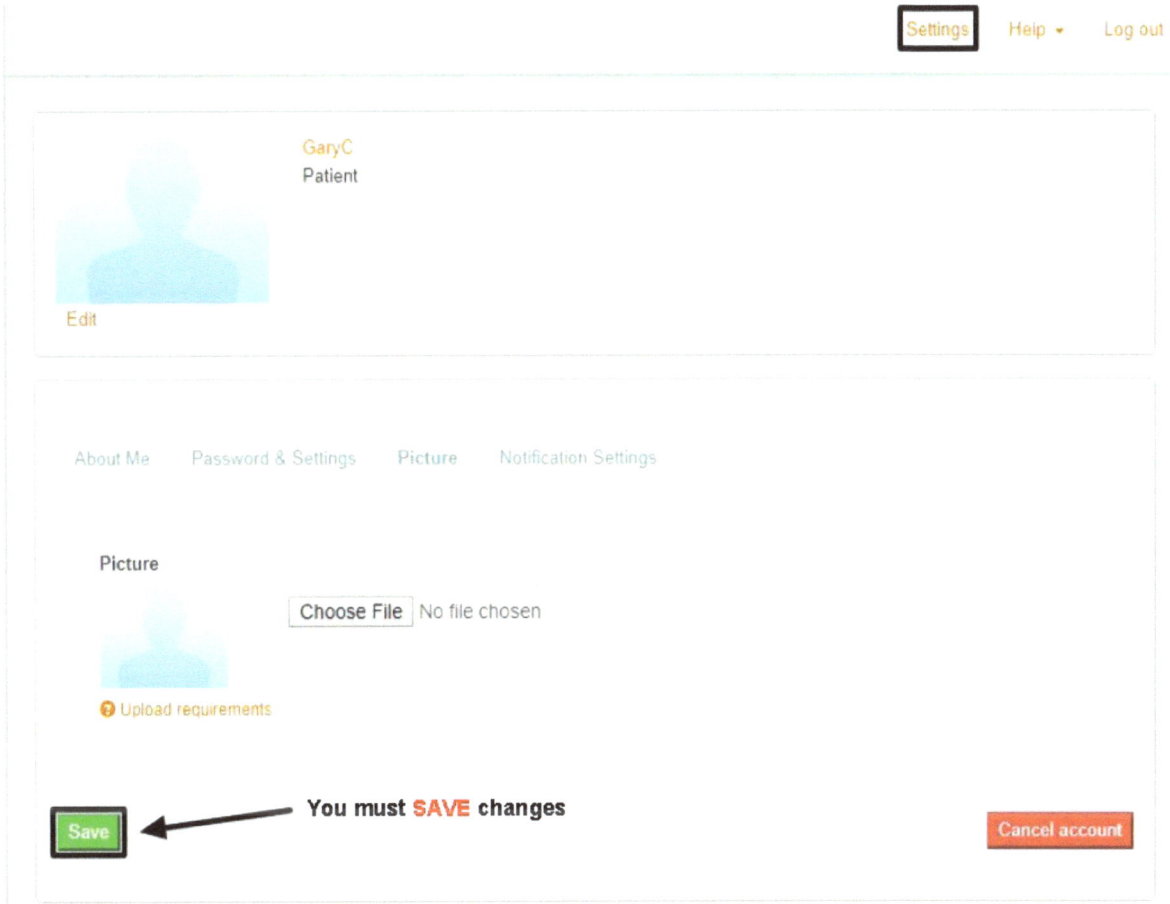

Notifications Page

Also in the Settings page, you can control which notifications and messages are emailed to you. Read these carefully. Then check the boxes you want to use. Then click on **Save**.

> *"As a working caregiver for my son, I love that I get notified about blogs here. And I can use the search box to find blogs that pertain to stuff my son is dealing with."*
> — Caregiver/Dad To 28-Year-Old With Bone Sarcoma

Settings   Help ▾   Log out

GaryC
Patient

Edit

About Me   Password & Settings   Picture   **Notification Settings**

Contact settings

☑ Personal contact form

Comment follow-up notification settings

☐ Receive content follow-up notification e-mails

Receive comment follow-up notification e-mails

No notifications ▾

Check this box to receive e-mail notification for follow-up comments to comments you posted. You can later disable this on a post-by-post basis... so if you leave this to YES, you can still disable follow-up notifications for comments you don't want follow-up mails anymore - i.e. for very popular posts.

☑ Bridge Plan Comments

☑ Community Notices

☑ Blog Notifications

Save   You must **SAVE** changes   Cancel account

83

Deleting Accounts

If you wish to delete your account, you may do that in Settings. You will need your current password to do this.

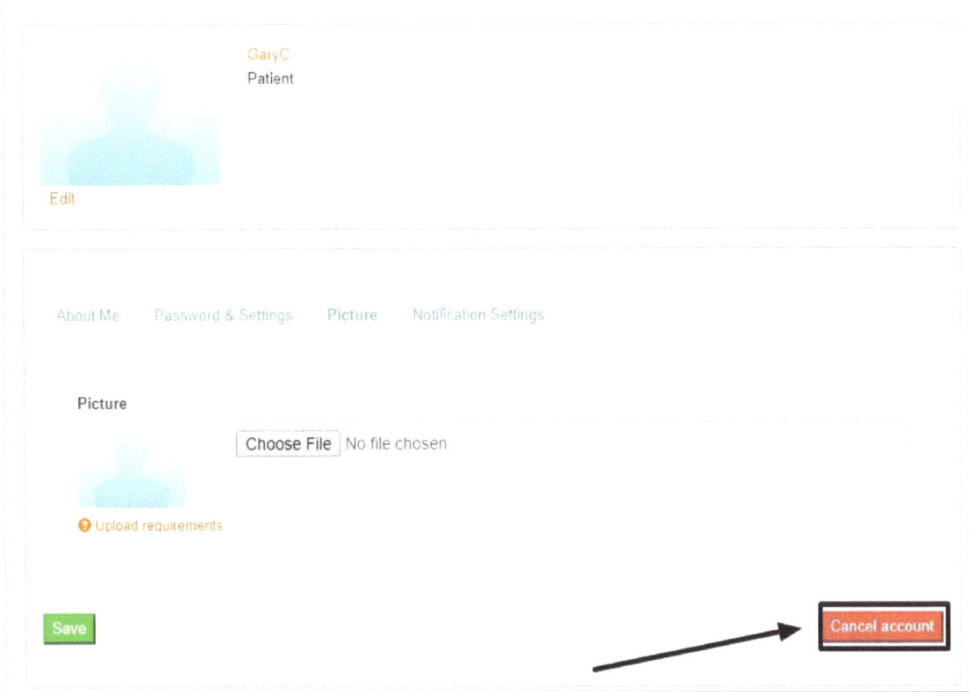

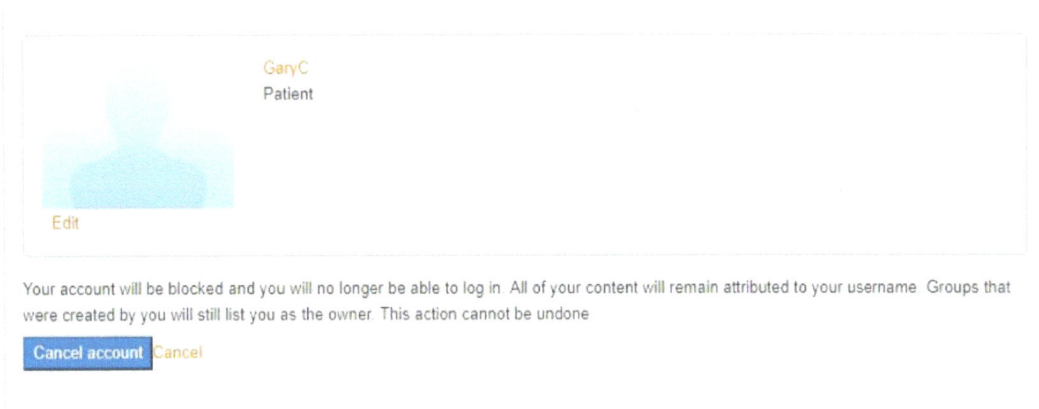

Your Landing Page

The My Bridge Plan is your landing page when you are logged in. Be sure to Bookmark this page. You can stayed logged in and always return to your place. Or if you log out, you will return to the Login page.

GCarstens
Patient

Edit

Diagnosis **1**   Treatment **1**   Healing **0**   Wellbeing **0**

This phase begins with your Diagnosis and ends when the decision is made on the first course of treatment. Set Health Goals for this phase and work with your Community to achieve them.

Diagnosis Goals   Add Goal+

                                                    Inspiring Image

Edit | Delete | ☑

Sleep

Get 8 hours of sleep a night by getting in bed by 10
good sleep will improve my condition.

2 comments | Add Comment

Username★   Log in

Enter your Reimagine Well Community username.

Password★

Enter the password that accompanies your username.

Log in   Forget Your Password?

Forgot your username or password? You can have a temporary password emailed to you.

SETTING ACHIEVABLE HEALTH GOALS

Understanding That It Works In Phases

Your Bridge Plan allows you to divide your own or your loved one's journey into phases. With the help of your community, ideally including your Care Team, you can set achievable health Goals for each phase of the journey.

Whether an individual is reeling from a recent diagnosis, or making the difficult transition from treatment into healing, achievable health goals are important. Life seems to make more sense - and give us a purpose - when we have a Goal.

> *"I have found the information here to be invaluable. Particularly the emphasis on goals… and the need to proactively deal with our disease."*
>
> *— 27-Year-Old With Soft Tissue Sarcoma*

GCarstens
Patient

Edit

Diagnosis **2**   Treatment **1**   Healing **0**   Wellbeing **0**

This phase begins with your Diagnosis and ends when the decision is made on the first course of treatment. Set Health Goals for this phase and work with your Community to achieve them.

Diagnosis Goals

Add Goal+

Edit | Delete | ☐

Healthy Eating

My new goal is to eat more fruits and vegetables, and limit how much I eat out every week. Also I need to avoid heavily processed foods and soda intake, so I can work my way to a healthy weight.

0 comments | Add Comment

Inspiring Image

Edit

Edit | Delete | ☑

Sleep

Get 8 hours of sleep a night by getting in bed by 10 PM to wake up at 6 AM. I know that getting good sleep will improve my condition.

2 comments | Add Comment

Setting Achievable Health Goals For Each Phase

Goals are the heart of anyone's Bridge Plan. Setting Goals establishes a vision of your future. Adding Goals to your Bridge Plan enables your support community to hold you accountable, as well as knowing how to best support you and help you achieve those goals. Knowing they have your back will give you strength. If you are a caregiver, and your patient is mature enough to help guide his or her own journey, this would be a great place to work together with them on setting these health Goals.

"My goal is to use my inner strength and find comfort from my family, friends, and medical team!"

— 18-Year-Old With Leukemia

Add Goals that will move you or your patient toward the next phase of their journey.

Make your Goals as clean, clear, specific, time-bound, and measurable as you can.

For example:

"Confirm on Sunday who will be picking my daughter up from daycare Monday, Wednesday, and Thursday as I go through my fertility tests with my doctor."

"Work out a schedule with my boss so I can work remotely from the hospital during Thursday infusions."

"Connect with three Bridge Builders who are also dealing with Oncofertility issues who are one phase ahead of me and can advise me during this time."

"Go with my class to the planetarium Monday and make it a "don't say the C word" day!"

"Go biking with my son both weekend days for one entire month to get exercise, before he has his cancer surgery. Then, reset this Goal for his healing phase."

Here is a great blog on how to set achievable health goals: www.reimaginewellcommunity.com/weblog/setting-health-goals

Completing Goals

Setting achievable health goals, and completing them, will help you continue to feel like you are moving forward. When you complete a Goal, check the box that is beside it and watch your completion graph grow! Your community of friends can tell how you are doing, and can encourage you in the Comment section.

> *"The support can save your life! If you're confused and scared about your cancer diagnosis, then this is a good place to start on your journey to recovery."*
>
> — *23-Year-Old With Brain Cancer*

Instructions:
1. Check your Goals when you complete them.
2. Once you have completed all Goals in a Phase, your progress bar will be complete.
3. When someone leaves a Goal comment, you will be notified by email. (You can remove this feature in Profile settings)
4. As you complete Goals, don't forget to celebrate your victories, large and small.

Motivation Keeps You Going

It's not just the cheers and hoorays from the members of your community that will keep you going. You need other motivations to continue to move forward. Reward yourself with healthy treats, some new clothes, a book or music download you've always wanted. Think about that trip to a National Park or Hawaii you've always dreamed about. Even something simple will do, like walking through a beautiful garden.

Celebrate the good things and people in your life. Send doctors who've helped you a thank you note. Let a friendly social worker know how you're doing. Thank friends who have always been there for you. These things can be rewarding, and motivating, too!

What And Who Are Your Powerful Motivators?

Think about what else in life motivates you, excites you and gives you an emotional lift. It might be family, friends, teachers, classmates or coworkers. Who are people that rooted and cheered for you? Imagine their faces. Use these memories to keep you going.

"Have something in your hands… a scrapbook with photos… it's such a motivational thing to have something you can feel and touch… to remind you this is why we're doing these things."
— Grandparent To A 17-Year-Old With Testicular Cancer

Gather Photos To Inspire You

Photos inspire you, and can be especially uplifting and powerful if you need some help to get through your day. Think about the photos you have on your desk, on your computer screen saver at school or work, on your favorite social media sites, and on your phone.

Find photos to make you laugh, smile, and glad to be alive. Add "Inspiring Pictures" to your Bridge Plan for you and your community members to see.

Diagnosis 1   Treatment 1   Healing 0   Wellbeing 0

This phase ends with the completion of the initial treatment. Be sure to engage your Community on setting and achieving yo
Treatment Health Goals.

Treatment Goals

Edit | Delete | ✔

Sleeping Well

Get 8 hours of sleep a night by getting in bed by 10 PM to wake up at 6 AM. I know that getting good sleep will improve my condition.

1 comment   Add Comment

Inspiring Image
Add Picture

Instructions:
- Choose <u>Add</u> in the Inspiring Picture box.
- Choose Phase from drop down menu.
- Choose a picture file (32mb or less) from your computer.
- Wait for the picture to upload, then <u>Save</u>.

Create Inspiring Image - Treatment

Inspiring Treatment

Choose File | No file chosen

❷ Upload requirements

Save

Upload requirements

- One file only.
- 32 MB limit.
- Allowed types: png, gif, jpg, jpeg

Create Inspiring Image - Treatment   ✕

Inspiring Treatment

Sally 1.png   903.42 KB
Remove

Save

Learn to Tell Your Story

Sharing the story of your life, whether you are a patient or a caregiver, as you go through diagnosis, treatment, healing, and wellbeing, can be extremely helpful. You may not know it now, but your story will help and inspire others. It will give them a glimpse into the truth of your life experiences. It may also give them hope to overcome their own challenges.

Sharing your story - and commenting in a helpful way on the stories of others - is one more good way we have of learning we are not alone. There are Comment buttons in several places on your Bridge Plan. These allow you and your community members to interact. Connect. Comment. And help one another build Bridge Plans.

The Best...

Treatment

Hello Everyone! I hope that sharing my story will help someone out there going through the same thing I am.

I am at the moment recovered from double mastectomy and am pretty proud of myself for recuperating so fast, even the doctors are amazed! So my advice for a speedy recovery is keep healthy excercise every day. Its hard but in the end it really helps!

The hardest thing since being diagnosed with breast cancer is how much of a surprise it was, my husband and I have been married for almost two years, we were just getting settled into our new life, and were thinking of trying to have a baby. It overwhelmed me to think that my right to give life was gone in instant, everyone around us were giving us the reality checks, chemo would render me infertile, its to late to start any fertility treatments because it takes too long, you need to start chemo now because being so young your cancer can be so agressive, and on top of that because I was BRCA 2 positive my kids had 50% chance of having my cancer gene. I cried my eyes out so many times, it hurt so much to think that I wasn't normal that all around me my friends where having babies and I wanted to have that ...it was hard really hard accepting the fact that I would never have kids.

But than I had an amazing friend who encouraged me, researched for me, and gave us hope ...we could be parents, through the amazing technology today we could have a baby that could be cancer free and freeze my eggs until I was ready. My husband and I were excited! But than boom they hit us with the price $8,000 dollars up front that my medical insurance could not cover. I was devastated my husband and I knew that we couldn't afford that, and again I resigned myself to not having kids. You don't even know how much decisions like this affect your mental state, I was soo tired every day, and not even thinking that the overwhelming fact that I was going to be infertile and never have a chance to have even one child. But, I knew that I was blessed blessed to have had survived what I had already been through and was looking onward to getting thru chemo and moving forward with living life to its max!

And than my dearest friend called again, she filled me with hope again and did one of the greatest things for us ...she along with friends, family, strangers, and facebook, raised the money for us to start the very costly fertility treatments. My husband and I had prayed for the right decision, and it came in such an amazing way thru the support of friends, family, and strangers! You cannot even comprehend the overwhelming sense of gratitude every time we received checks in the mail and still are from friends from all over the world who cared enough to donate.

I am currently undergoing the fertility treatments, and I do not like needles, and I have to get a shot every day, but each prick reminds me that my amazing friends and family make me an AMAZING SURVIVOR! I have hope hope for a better tomorrow and boy am I reminded every day that I am not going to die! I have way too much to live for! So I am going to fight! Fight for what I can achieve and live for many tomorrows! lol!

So what better way than to stay positive, life is short but living now is living for so much more! So I am a survivor and although chemo does not sound good....I am blessed blessed that there have been so many others that have gone through what I have gone through and survived to know that I can too, and now more than ever because I now know that I have a future to share with my husband and that future little possibility that I still have the right to give life, and hope to others that are going through what I am going through.

> *"We should always be willing to share our stories with the newly diagnosed, and to be a calming influence. Challenge them to make informed decisions!"*
> — 32-Year-Old With Spinal Cord Tumors

Building Your Team

So you've begun your Bridge Plan. You've posted information about yourself. You've written some achievable health Goals. You've invited trusted people into your community, and added photos that motivate you. You've learned how to tell your story so other Bridge Builders - that is, other patients, caregivers, and family members who are part of the Reimagine Well Support Community - will read it, understand it, and relate to it.

Maybe some of them have already begun to support you. And maybe some family members, friends, or members of your Care Team whom you've invited to be with you on your journey have begun to support you as well.

Always Surround Yourself With Love And Support

Think of your Reimagine Well Support Community as your "health family." You need people like that, who'll surround you with love and support. People who can understand and relate to what you've been through. Some of them may become your mentors, and some of them may be mentored by YOU.

Just like real life.

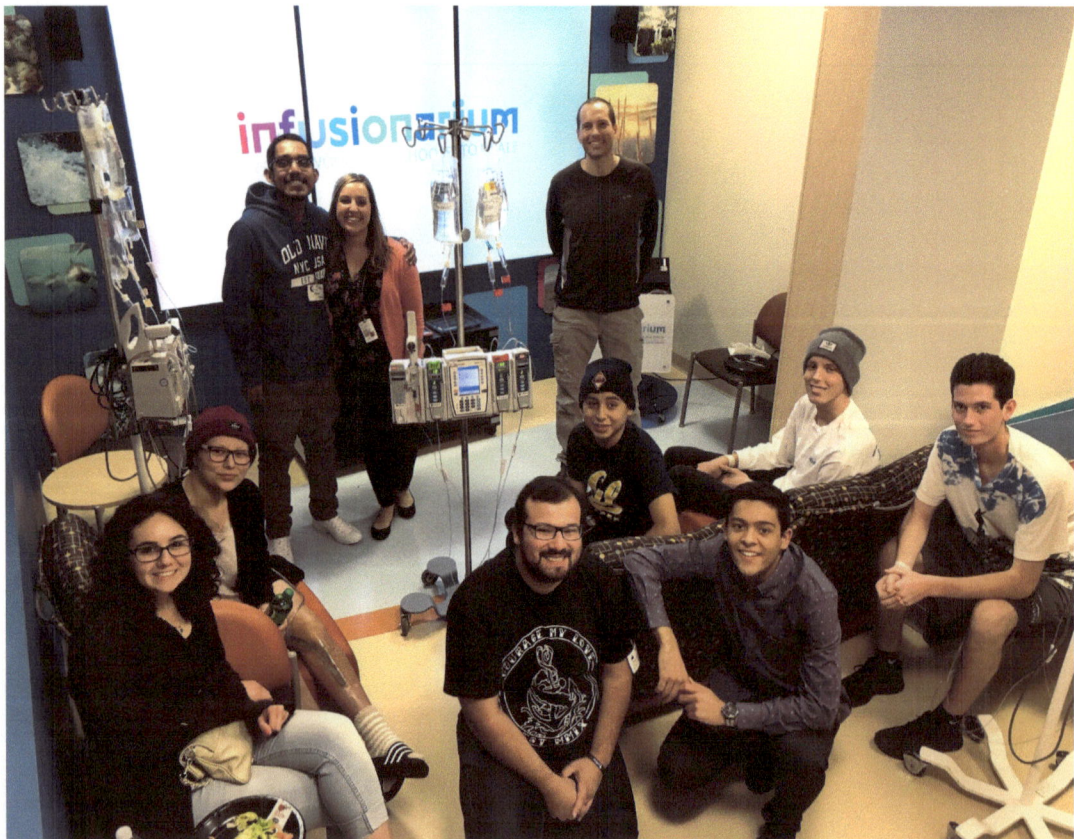

Making a Safe, Supportive Community For Yourself

The Reimagine Well Support Community is a place to gather your strongest allies. You can unite them to become an integrated part of the next step in your journey. You can use the My Community button to send invitations, and keep up with requests you've sent and received. Everyone in your Community will automatically receive email updates when you post or comment on your blog(s).

> *"Find a way to have fun… laugh and smile, and bring people around you who'll allow you to laugh and smile."*
>
> — *18-Year-Old With Osteosarcoma*

Instructions:
1. Don't forget to scroll down to check your Share wall.
2. Share comments are limited to 750 characters.
3. When someone posts a comment in your Share wall you will be notified by email. (You can remove this feature in Profile settings)

Check Out The Suggested Community Members

Use the Suggested Community Members tool to connect with other Bridge Builders. These are people with whom you have a lot in common. This can be a lifesaver - there is someone who understands what you've been through.

Take a moment to read about the cancer journey experiences and suggestions of others.

The first time you do this, give yourself a little time. Like any other new social media platform, you may find yourself "falling down the rabbit hole."

A few hours later, you're gonna look up and say, "These people get me!"

Community Requests   Email Invites

My Community Requests

👤 My Community 8

Community Requests 0

Email Invites

❤ Tips 4 Life
    Favorite Tips 0
    Write Tips

Invite Friends

Email★

☑ Infusionarium
    Immersive Healing Experiences 3
    Learn Guides 1

Email subject★

GCarstens has sent you an invite!

Email Message★

📰 My Blog 0

📄 My Notes

Send Invitation

Instructions:
1.   From Community Requests open Email Invites.
2.   You can invite one person at a time. Type in their email address and your personal message, then click Send Invitation.

My Bridge Plan

My Community 7
Community Requests 0

Tips 4 Life
Favorite Tips 0
Write Tips

Infusionarium
Immersive Healing Experiences 3
Learn Guides 1

My Blog 0

My Notes

Print Bridge Book

My Community

Sort by   Recently Active ⌄   Order   Desc ⌄

Miami Cancer Institute
Miami Cancer Institute
Cancer
Healthcare
Professional
Remove User

Roger - Co-Founder
Cancer (Thyroid)
Patient
Remove User

Reim...
Comm...
Healt...
Profe...
Remo...

My Bridge 4 Life
Healthcare
Professional
Remove User

Ryan Callahan
Cancer (Breast)
Supporter / Caregiver
Remove User

Suggested Community Members

zshihab
Anxiety Disorder
Patient

Add User   Next»

CONNECT WITH OTHER MEMBERS

Suggested Community Members

zshihab
Anxiety Disorder
Patient

Add User   Next»

CONNECT WITH OTHER MEMBERS

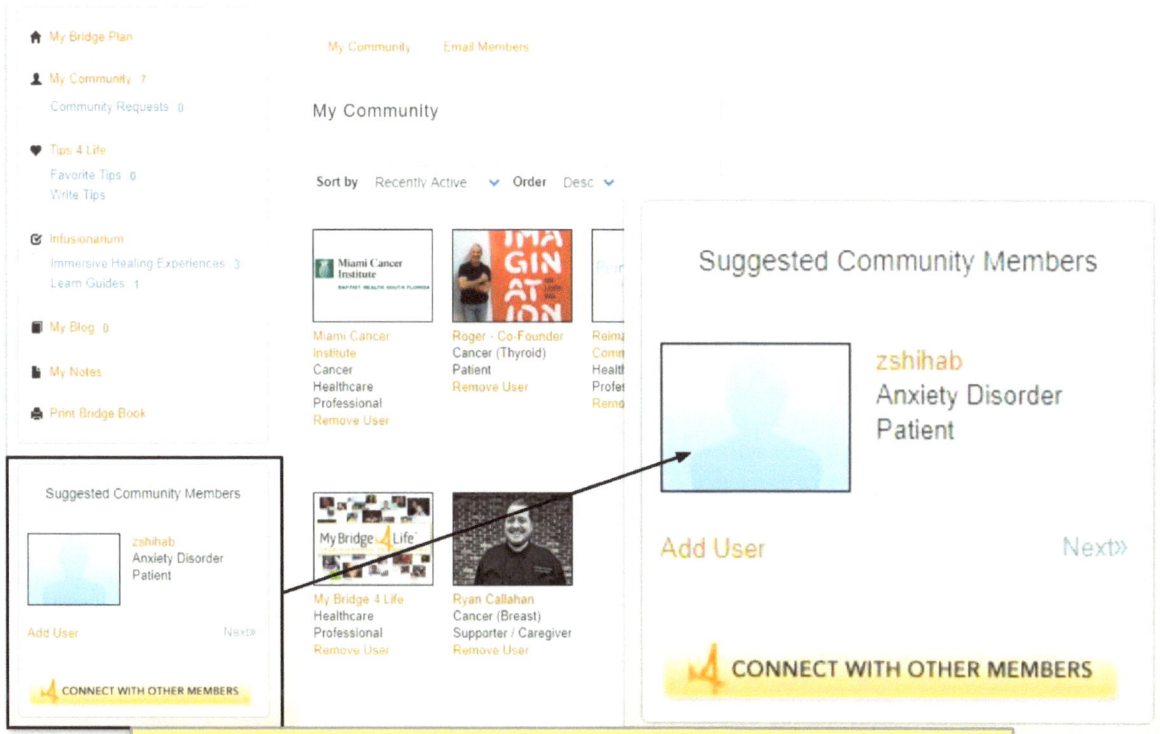

Instructions:

1. The Suggested Community Members box will display other Bridge Builders, starting with those who share what you are "Dealing With".
2. Use the Add User button to send them a community request.
3. Use Next to scroll through the suggestions.

98

Find Your Tribe: The Benefits of Support Groups

It is important for you to communicate with people who understand you and what you are going through. We call that "Finding Your Tribe."

There's another way to find Bridge Builders to add to your Community. It's the Connect With Other Members button. You can even filter other Bridge Builders by Illness, Condition, Phase, Role, and Location. Find Your Tribe!

Instructions:
1. Use the Connect with Other Members button to take you to this page.
2. Use the checkboxes to filter.
3. The more filters you set, the smaller the number of Bridge Builders you'll get.
4. Use the Add User buttons, one Bridge Builder at a time, to send community requests.

Other Support Organizations

When you first join, you may have only one or two Support Organizations in My Community. An easy way to find other Bridge Builders and Support Organizations is to visit their Bridge Plans. You will see their members. And you can send requests to them.

So that you know… accepting a community request is optional. Meaning it's not required by you, or by the person to whom you send a request.

Instructions:
1. Start in My Community, click on any Hospital or Support Organization.
2. Use the Add User buttons that you see below members' pictures to send a request to join their Community.
3. You can also look at the Community of anyone in your Community for Bridge Builders and Organizations to Add.

My Blog and Commenting On Another's Blog

My Blog allows you to publicly share about your journey. Your community will be told when you post a new blog; it's an easy way to communicate. Blog posts are searchable by our global community via tags, keywords, and illness/condition.

REMEMBER: Blogs (and other postings) are all reviewed by our medical staff and/or the National Institutes of Health before they are published. It may take up to 48 hours to see your blog in the feed. And if there are responses to your blog that you feel are objectionable, you may delete them.

"Beginning the process, telling my story, going back to explore, each step has been therapeutic! Through my blog, I give a voice to my journey and emotions."
— Parent To A 22-Year-Old With Uterine Sarcoma

Instructions:
1. Choose Add a New Blog Post.
2. Pick a title, Phase, and write your Blog post.
3. You can attach files to your Blog. Look for File Attachments below the text box and above the Save button.
4. Select Save and your Blog is created. (It will be reviewed before it is published and usually takes 24-48 hours)
5. Your Community members will be notified by email once it's published.
6. Community members can leave comments on your Blog post.
7. You can delete comments.
8. You can Edit or Delete your Blog.

To comment on another Bridge Builder's blog, look at the bottom of the blog. You'll find a Comment box. Enter a subject and your message. Then click the Save button. It will post but you will not see it immediately. It often takes a few moments for the comment to make its way through the administration server. The Blogger will receive an email notifying them about the comment, as will others who have commented.

"Coming Out" In Public, Social Media, Blogging

One more suggestion before we move on to other uses you can make of your Bridge Plan.

"Coming out" to others about a cancer journey, no matter what phase of it you are in, and whether you are a patient or a caregiver, is a brave and often difficult thing to do.

Roger Holzberg, Reimagine Well's co-founder, and an adult cancer survivor, says it can be very complicated. Especially during diagnosis and treatment. There are so many people to keep up on what's currently happening. He recommends to newly diagnosed patients and their caregivers that they consider "what they expect" from those they tell during early phases, and communicate that information clearly to those people.

For many of us, sharing every detail of your life on Facebook, Twitter, Instagram, and other social media is just another part of daily life. That's not always true for members of older generations, who didn't grow up with social media.

However you feel about this, just remember whatever you decide to do publicly - let it all hang out or keep it close to the vest - understand that **what you post in your Bridge Plan will only be accessible to the people you accept into your Reimagine Well community.**

These people and you will share something in common. They will be supporters and your allies. If you want to try out new thoughts or ideas about your illness with them first, it would be a great place to start. Then, as Dr. Sender says, "Go tell the world."

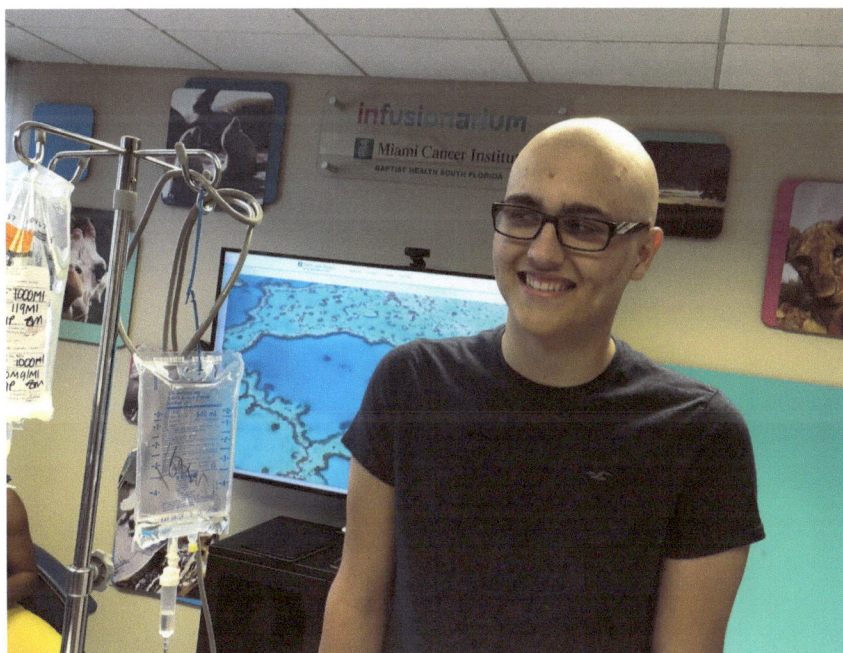

Notes

Notes

Keeping Organized

Start With Medical Contact Information

Use your Medical Contacts to keep track of contact information for fertility specialists, pediatric social workers, oncology genetic counselors, physical therapists, registered dietitians and other medical professionals with whom you've come in contact.

Under your Medical Notes you can keep an organized record of other important information, too. This can include post-appointment doctor summaries, details about medications and dosage, and needed advice from any Care Team members. After treatment is over, you can use your End of Treatment Summary to get this information. You may also include pathology reports and other info you feel is important.

PLEASE BE AWARE: In order to protect medical information and insure its privacy, none of the medical information on this page is able to be shared publicly. If you'd like to share something with your community, you will need to enter it in your public blog.

Recording Post-Appointment Summaries, Medications and Dosages, Advice From Medical Professionals And Support Groups

Below are instructions on how to keep track of the medical professionals with whom you have interacted. You can also record medical notes and other information here.

Again, medical information is always private. It can only be seen by you, unless you print it out and show the printed paper to someone.

My Notes

Use Contacts to keep track of any contact information for healthcare providers, organizations, community members, etc. Under your Notes you can keep an organized record of any other important information, such as post-appointment summaries, advice from medical professionals and community members, or next steps and reminders.

IMPORTANT: In order to protect your personal information and insure its privacy, none of the information on this page will be shared publicly. If you'd like to share any of the information on this page, you will need to enter it in your public Blog

Diagnosis   Treatment   Healing   Wellbeing

Contacts

Add Contact   Help

Edit | Delete
Dr. Shawn Veiseh
1 (310) 794-7940
Corporate Physical Program

Instructions and Guidance:
1. Select My Notes tab to open the page.
2. Use the Add button to enter doctors, healthcare providers, and any other sources you feel are important places you go to facilitate your health.
3. Phase by Phase, use this space to document private things that you do not want to share with your larger community in your Notes.

Notes

Add Note   Help

Edit | Delete
My Medical Notes

Personal Notes: It's really frustrating that I don't even know if I have cancer or not. I am REFUSING to believe that my life is in jeopardy - I will not let that in. I am still going to the gym every day and building up my stamina and inner strength. I have started walking up to the top of the hill near my house at sunrise and greeting the sun with a prayer for the dawning of the day. I hate that I have not yet told my kids, but I do not want to burden them! My Dad has really stepped up to the plate and is totally supporting me, and my delay in the surgery.

Edit | Delete
My Medical Notes

A physician/acquaintance warned me against using diagnosis tools (like an MRI) because it can show a lot of 'false positives.' For me, chasing a few 'false positives' was well worth the early detection of finding the one REAL positive – get a great physician to read and interpret the data.

Tips 4 Life - From And For Others

Tips 4 Life is a global database of real-world wisdom for you and your loved ones - made by regular people and healthcare professionals who have been where you are now.

As you complete each phase of your cancer journey, we strongly encourage you to leave behind Tips 4 Life and Blogs for the people who are following in your footsteps.

Each time you want to check for new tips, click on My New Tips. That will open a window with the newest tips for the entire community. To find the relevant tips for you, select Filter Tips. After you use Filter Tips, My New Tips will open a window with the tips you have requested.

> *"Folks learn because the authors can add tags and they are searchable!"*
> — *Grandparent To A 23-Year-Old With Germ Cell Tumors*

Or you can begin by selecting an illness only, then clicking the Filter Tips button. Selecting additional filters will narrow your tip results. Remember to save your favorites. If you'd like to gain deeper knowledge about a tip from your favorites, click on the Bridge Builder's name to join their community. You can contact them directly with questions about their Tip 4 Life.

As you work through this section of the Bridge Plan, you'll find instructions about how to select your Favorite Tips, contact other Bridge Builders, write tips of your own and how to search through other Tips 4 Life and Blogs. In the Help section, there is also a full start-up guide with "Best Practices" available to download if necessary.

Immersive Healing Experiences

Reimagine Well's "immersive healing experiences" are requested/directed by patient vision teams at our partner institutions for use while in all phases of the patient journey, especially while in the treatment phase. Also featured are live events hosted by our partner hospitals, featuring a variety of special guests and experts.

Learn Guides Are Designed To Provide Education – 24/7 – Across The Entire Patient Journey

From diagnosis, to treatment, then on to healing and wellbeing. Learn Guides are rich media experiences with video, photos, resource links and much more. They can be downloaded as Ebooks on patient phones, tablets and computers, able to be used when and where they are needed.

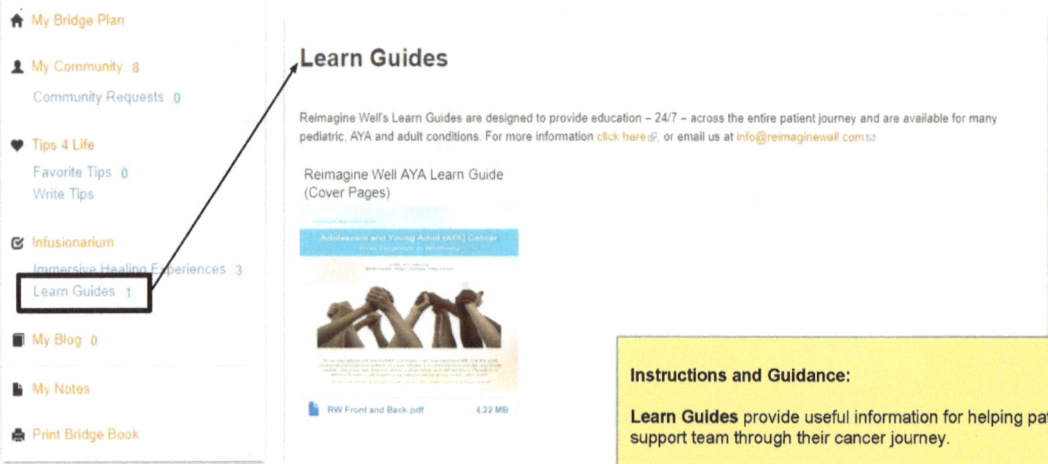

Instructions and Guidance:

Learn Guides provide useful information for helping patients and their support team through their cancer journey.

You can download any available **Learn Guides** on this page.

Print Your Bridge Book - Chronicle Of Your Journey

You can print out your Bridge Book. We encourage all Bridge Builders to print a copy of their Bridge Book after each phase of their journey. You should have it with you at all meetings - whether you are a patient or a caregiver - that you have with your Care Team.

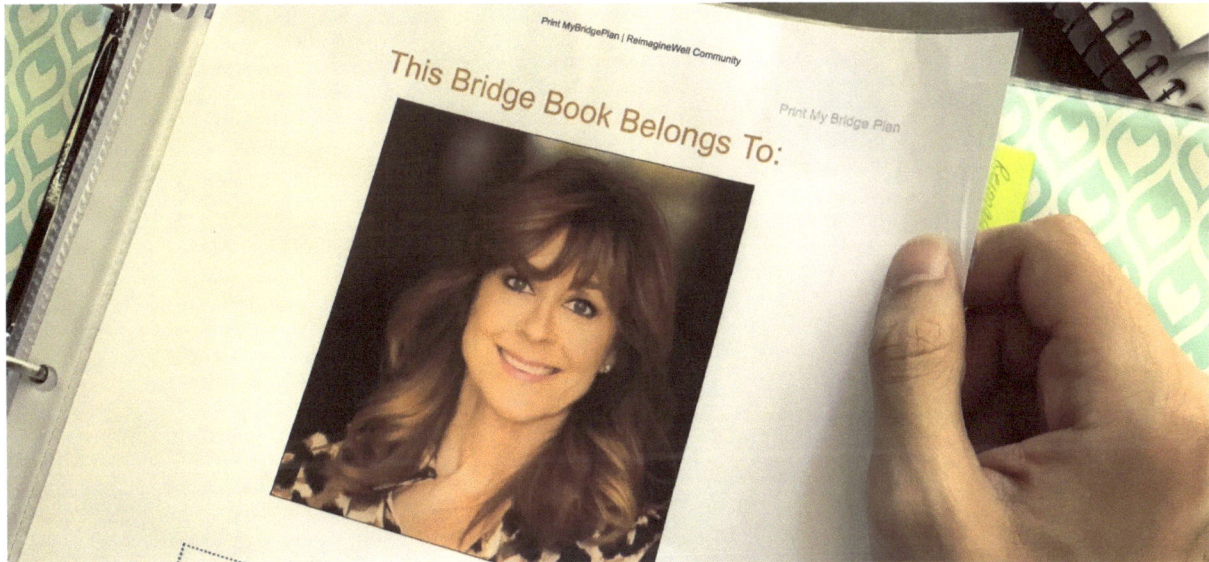

Your printed Bridge Book becomes a chronicle of your journey, from Diagnosis through Treatment, Healing, and on to Wellbeing. Many Bridge Builders and Parents print them out, bind them, and keep a copy on the coffee table or bookshelf.

Notes

Healing And Moving Forward

As Dr. Sender said at the beginning of Part Two of this Learn Guide, "You have to become empowered to ask the right questions, and to find the right questions to get the information you need." In other words, Knowledge Is Power.

Resources For Healing and Moving Forward

There are many resources available for you and your caregivers. This Learn Guide is full of links to reputable and reliable organizations whom you can trust, specifically the National Institutes of Health, the National Cancer Institute and the American Cancer Society. You should feel free to roam around their websites, along with the links below.

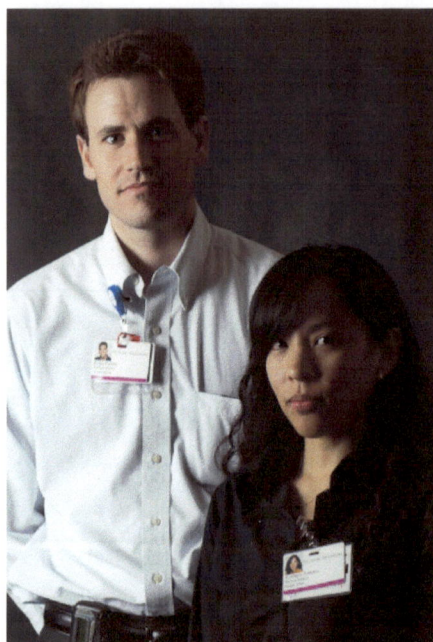

TO LEARN MORE

Setting Health Goals: https://www.reimaginewellcommunity.com/node/7623

National Institutes of Health: https://www.nih.gov/

National Cancer Institute: https://www.cancer.gov/

American Cancer Society: https://www.cancer.org/

NCI Office of Survivorship - Resources: https://cancercontrol.cancer.gov/ocs/resources/survivors.html

Cancer Survivors Managing Their Health: https://bit.ly/2lirn7K

Cancer Survivorship Research: https://bit.ly/2wqVeQf

Coping With Cancer Survivorship: https://www.cancer.gov/about-cancer/coping/survivorship

NCI - A Tough Transition to Cancer Survivorship: https://www.cancer.gov/about-cancer/coping/research/survivorship-plans

Being A Mentor

Mentoring is a process in which you share your experiences with another patient or caregiver. Often this is an individual who is experiencing what you have already gone through. By mentoring them, you empower them. The same way you were empowered. You give them hope. And you strengthen them for what lies ahead. You can mentor others by volunteering at the hospital where you or your loved one was treated, or your own local hospital or medical center. You can help in an online community or by phone. Giving back not only helps another person, it helps you, as well.

Getting Mentored

You or your caregiver might feel as if you need a mentor. Someone to help you through whatever phase you are in now.

There are many places where you can go to find someone to talk to, and perhaps even spend some time with. These services do exist. As the expression goes: help is just a phone call away. You'll find a list of links to these services below.

"Every cancer survivor is a researcher. As you communicate your treatment and what you have been through, your doctors will continue to learn and use this knowledge to treat the patients who follow you. So, don't stop communicating – your doctors always learn and adapt treatment based on the knowledge that they gain from you!"

— Lilibeth Torno, M.D.

TO LEARN MORE

Organizations & Resources to Support Young Cancer Patients: https://www.cancer.gov/types/aya

4th Angel – Patient & Caregiver Mentoring Program: http://www.4thangel.org/

Cancer Connects Volunteer Mentor Program: http://www.cancerconnects.org/volunteerMentorProgram

Imerman Angels: http://imermanangels.org/

Notes

The Future

As we told you on the first page of this Learn Guide, stop and take a breath. Let it out, long and slow. Look around you. Look behind you. Look forward.

That's the way you are heading now. Straight into your, or your loved one's, future.

Illness has a way of focusing people. It makes them see, hear, and feel what is really important. What matters. What counts.

A walk down a country road in the fall, as the leaves are glowing a bright red and gold.   A July 4th dinner with your family, one where everyone gets along. Watching the sun set over the ocean, a lake, or even a glacier.

Getting together with friends you love, and who love you back. Hugging those friends and telling them, "Thank you for being there for me." And then turning around and being there for them when they need you.

Life, it is said, can be wonderful, awful, strange, funny, and familiar, all at the same time. It can also be hard and frustrating, glorious and awesome.

If you're reading this, you're imagining a brighter tomorrow.
That's what is important.
That's what matters.
That's what counts.

You have been deepened, broadened, and strengthened by your journey. You have grown. You're a different person now. And you're not alone. Take one more deep breath.

Then start walking straight into your well-earned future.

> *"Keep healthy. Keep your spirit up. Live every day to the fullest!"*
> *—18-Year-Old With Lymphoma*

Notes

Glossary

Adoption *(uh-dop-shuh n)*	Adoption is a process whereby a person assumes the parenting of another, usually a child, from that person's biological or legal parent or parents, and, in so doing, permanently transfers all rights and responsibilities, along with filiation, from the biological parent or parents.
Alkylating agent *(AL-kuh-LAY-ting AY-jent)*	A type of drug that is used in the treatment of cancer. It interferes with the cell's DNA and inhibits cancer cell growth.
Cardiovascular *(KAR-dee-oh-VAS-kyoo-ler)*	Having to do with the heart and blood vessels.
Cervical cancer *(SER-vih-kul KAN-ser)*	Cancer that forms in tissues of the cervix (the organ connecting the uterus and vagina). It is usually a slow-growing cancer that may not have symptoms but can be found with regular Pap tests (a procedure in which cells are scraped from the cervix and looked at under a microscope). Cervical cancer is almost always caused by human papillomavirus (HPV) infection.
Chemotherapy *(KEE-moh-THAYR-uh-pee)*	Treatment that uses drugs to stop the growth of cancer cells, either by killing the cells or by stopping them from dividing. Chemotherapy may be given by mouth, injection, or infusion, or on the skin, depending on the type and stage of the cancer being treated. It may be given alone or with other treatments, such as surgery, radiation therapy, or biologic therapy.
Contraception *(KON-truh-SEP-shun)*	The use of drugs, devices, or surgery to prevent pregnancy. There are many different types of contraception. These include barrier methods to keep sperm from fertilizing the egg, hormone methods, intrauterine devices (IUDs), and surgery to close the fallopian tubes in women or close off the two tubes that carry sperm out of the testicles in men. Also called birth control.
Cryopreservation *(KRY-oh-PREH-zer-VAY-shun)*	The process of cooling and storing cells, tissues, or organs at very low or freezing temperatures to save them for future use. Also called cryobanking.
DNA	The molecules inside cells that carry genetic information and pass it from one generation to the next. Also called deoxyribonucleic acid.
Fertility *(fer-TIH-lih-tee)*	The ability to produce children.
Fertility preservation *(fer-TIH-lih-tee PREH-zer-VAY-shun)*	A type of procedure used to help keep a person's ability to have children. A fertility preservation procedure is done before a medical treatment that may cause infertility, such as radiation therapy or chemotherapy. Examples of fertility preservation procedures include sperm banking, egg freezing, in vitro fertilization with embryo freezing, and certain types of surgery for cervical and ovarian cancer.

119

Hematologic Cancer *(HEE-muh-tuh-LAH-jik KAN-ser*	Cancer that begins in blood-forming tissue, such as the bone marrow, or in the cells of the immune system. Examples of hematologic cancer are leukemia, lymphoma, and multiple myeloma. Also called blood cancer.
Hormonal Therapy *(hor-MOH-nul THAYR-uh-pee)*	Treatment that adds, blocks, or removes hormones. For certain conditions (such as diabetes or menopause), hormones are given to adjust low hormone levels. Hormones can cause certain cancers (such as prostate and breast cancer) to grow. To slow or stop the growth of cancer, synthetic hormones or other drugs may be given to block the body's natural hormones. Sometimes surgery is needed to remove the gland that makes a certain hormone. Also called endocrine therapy, hormone therapy, and hormone treatment.
Hormone *(HOR-mone)*	One of many substances made by glands in the body. Hormones circulate in the bloodstream and control the actions of certain cells or organs. Some hormones can also be made in the laboratory.
Infertile *(in-FER-til)*	Unable to produce children.
Malignant *(muh-LIG-nunt)*	Cancerous. Malignant cells can invade and destroy nearby tissue and spread to other parts of the body.
Menstruation *(MEN-stroo-WAY-shun)*	Periodic discharge of blood and tissue from the uterus. From puberty until menopause, menstruation occurs about every 28 days when a woman is not pregnant.
Oncology *(on-KAH-loh-jee)*	A branch of medicine that specializes in the diagnosis and treatment of cancer. It includes medical oncology (the use of chemotherapy, hormone therapy, and other drugs to treat cancer), radiation oncology (the use of radiation therapy to treat cancer), and surgical oncology (the use of surgery and other procedures to treat cancer).
Oocyte Cryopreservation *(OH-oh-site KRY-oh-PREH-zer-VAY-shun)*	The process of freezing one or more unfertilized eggs (eggs that have not been combined with sperm) to save them for future use. The eggs are thawed and fertilized in the laboratory to make embryos that can be placed in a woman's uterus. Oocyte cryopreservation is being studied as a type of fertility preservation. It may be useful for women with cancer who want to have children after having radiation therapy, chemotherapy, or certain types of surgery, which can cause infertility. Also called egg banking, egg cryopreservation, and egg freezing.
Ovarian Cancer *(oh-VAYR-ee-un KAN-ser)*	Cancer that forms in tissues of the ovary (one of a pair of female reproductive glands in which the ova, or eggs, are formed). Most ovarian cancers are either ovarian epithelial cancers (cancer that begins in the cells on the surface of the ovary) or malignant germ cell tumors (cancer that begins in egg cells). Fallopian tube cancer and primary peritoneal cancer are similar to ovarian epithelial cancer and are staged and treated the same way.

Ovarian *(oh-VAYR-ee-un)*	Having to do with the ovaries, the female reproductive glands in which the ova (eggs) are formed. The ovaries are located in the pelvis, one on each side of the uterus.
Ovarian Tissue Banking *(oh-VAYR-ee-un TIH-shoo BANK-ing)*	The process of freezing ovarian tissue to save for future infertility treatment. Part or all of an ovary is removed, and the tissue that contains the eggs is cut into thin slices and frozen. The tissue may later be thawed and placed back into the woman's body, usually on the remaining ovary. Ovarian tissue banking is a type of fertility preservation. It may be useful for women who want to have children after having treatment that may cause infertility, such as certain cancer treatments. Also called ovarian tissue cryopreservation and ovarian tissue freezing.
Pituitary Gland *(pih-TOO-ih-TAYR-ee)*	One of many substances made by glands in the body. Hormones circulate in the bloodstream and control the actions of certain cells or organs. Some hormones can also be made in the laboratory.
Premature Menopause *(PREE-muh-CHOOR MEH-nuh-pawz)*	A condition in which the ovaries stop working and menstrual periods stop before age 40. This can cause fertility problems and symptoms of menopause. There are two types of premature menopause, primary and secondary. Primary premature menopause means that the ovaries do not function normally. This may be because they have been removed by surgery, or it may be caused by some cancer treatments and certain diseases or genetic conditions. In secondary premature menopause, the ovaries are normal but there is a problem getting hormone signals to them from the brain. This is usually caused by diseases of the pituitary gland or hypothalamus. Some women with premature menopause sometimes have menstrual periods and may be able to have children. Also called early menopause, ovarian failure, and ovarian insufficiency.
Puberty *(PYOO-ber-tee)*	The time of life when a child experiences physical and hormonal changes that mark a transition into adulthood. The child develops secondary sexual characteristics and becomes able to have children. Secondary sexual characteristics include growth of pubic, armpit, and leg hair; breast enlargement; and increased hip width in girls. In boys, they include growth of pubic, face, chest and armpit hair; voice changes; penis and testicle growth, and increased shoulder width.
Radiation *(RAY-dee-AY-shun)*	Energy released in the form of particle or electromagnetic waves. Common sources of radiation include radon gas, cosmic rays from outer space, medical x-rays, and energy given off by a radioisotope (unstable form of a chemical element that releases radiation as it breaks down and becomes more stable). Radiation can damage cells. It is used to diagnose and treat some types of cancer.

Registered Dietitian *(dy-eh-TIH-shun)*	A health professional with special training in the use of diet and nutrition to keep the body healthy. A registered dietitian may help the medical team improve the nutritional health of a patient.
Reproductive System *(REE-proh-DUK-tiv SIS-tem)*	The organs involved in producing offspring. In women, this system includes the ovaries, the fallopian tubes, the uterus, the cervix, and the vagina. In men, it includes the prostate, the testes, and the penis.
Sperm *(spurm)*	The male reproductive cell, formed in the testicle. A sperm unites with an egg to form an embryo.
Surgery *(SER-juh-ree)*	A procedure to remove or repair a part of the body or to find out whether disease is present. An operation.
Surrogacy *(sur-uh-guh-see)*	The practice by which a woman (called a surrogate mother) becomes pregnant and gives birth to a baby in order to give it to someone who cannot have children.
Survivorship *(ser-VY-ver-ship)*	In cancer, survivorship focuses on the health and life of a person with cancer post treatment until the end of life. It covers the physical, psychosocial, and economic issues of cancer, beyond the diagnosis and treatment phases. Survivorship includes issues related to the ability to get health care and follow-up treatment, late effects of treatment, second cancers, and quality of life. Family members, friends, and caregivers are also considered part of the survivorship experience.
Testicle *(TES-tih-kul)*	One of two egg-shaped glands inside the scrotum that produce sperm and male hormones. Also called testis
Transplantation *(tranz-plan-TAY-shun)*	A surgical procedure in which tissue or an organ is transferred from one area of a person's body to another area, or from one person (the donor) to another person (the recipient).
Uterine Cancer *(YOO-teh-rin KAN-ser)*	Cancer that forms in tissues of the uterus (the small, hollow, pear-shaped organ in a woman's pelvis in which a fetus develops). Two types of uterine cancer are endometrial cancer (cancer that begins in cells lining the uterus) and uterine sarcoma (a rare cancer that begins in muscle or other tissues in the uterus).

"NCI Dictionary of Cancer Terms." National Cancer Institute, National Institutes of Health, https://www.cancer.gov/publications/dictionaries/cancer-terms

From Team Reimagine Well

"I've been involved with treating patients for nearly 30 years. The thing I want to say to a patient - and their caregivers - who has just completed treatment is, firstly, congratulations and, secondly, well done. What we need to talk about now is how we get you to your new normal, how we get you to adulthood, how we understand all the consequences of the therapy that you've been through, and how we make sure that you truly have wellness going forward."

— Leonard Sender, M.D.

"The new choices, options and opportunities for Fertility Preservation, along with new fertility treatments - even in the Survivorship period - that can be offered to patients has vastly expanded and increased in just the last five years!"

— Laxmi Kondapalli, M.D., MSCE

"I am a three-time cancer survivor. I had osteogenic sarcoma when I was 15, with two relapses, and I had ovarian cancer when I was 38. I hope that by seeing me "Get Busy Living," cancer patients have hope that it is possible to survive and thrive after cancer. It's also very important for me to help educate patients to become strong survivors."

— Jenee Areeckal, MSW, LCSW

"I love discussing Fertility Preservation with patients because it means that we are planning for their life beyond cancer. It is seen as a discussion of hope."

— Julie Messina, PA-C

"This is the time to nourish and nurture yourself. Take advantage of the resources that are available to help you make the best choices. When it comes to food and nutrition, reach out to a registered dietitian nutritionist. You will be in the hands of an expert who is trained to help you both deal with your journey to Wellbeing and Survivorship."

— Jocelyn Harrison, MPH, RD

"This is what The Bridge Plan is designed for. To enable and encourage mentoring and sharing wisdom. For me, it was nearly a year post-surgery before I was really ready to open up about the experience and share…. There will come a time when you look back on this with perspective and newfound knowledge. And you'll be celebrating milestones with your family for a long time to come. I'm sure of it!"

— Roger Holzberg, Cancer Survivor and Co-Founder Of Reimagine Well

Learn Guide Authors:

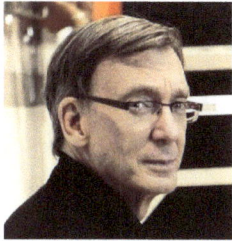

Martin Casella - Martin is an award-winning educator, playwright and screenwriter. He has taught writing at the California Institute of the Arts and at the Harvey Milk School, a NYC public high school with a focus on At Risk and LGBTQ students. At HMHS he created a writing program where teens learned to shape their life stories. The "What's Your Story" program now serves as a fundraising tool for the HMHS Student College Scholarship Fund. Martin has also written for Steven Spielberg, Kerry Washington, Lasse Hallstrom, Anthony Edwards, Whoopi Goldberg, John Milius, HBO, Disney, Universal, Warner Brothers and Paulist Productions. Among the writing awards he has won or been nominated for are The New York International Fringe Festival Overall Excellence Award for Playwriting (twice); the New York Outer Critics Circle for Best New Off-Broadway Musical; two GLAAD Award nominations for Outstanding New Play and Best New Off-Broadway Musical and LA WEEKLY Outstanding New Play Awards. Martin's plays are published by Samuel French and have been performed worldwide. He has written for Opera News, and his interactive writing credits include Steven Spielberg's Director's Chair.

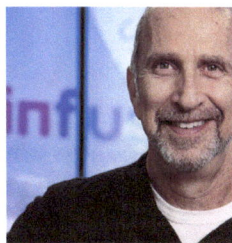

Roger Holzberg - Roger is the founder of My Bridge for Life™ and served as the first (consulting) Creative Director for the National Cancer Institute (NCI) where he led a multi-discipline Team to concept and build NCI's vision of how to educate patients, researchers, and healthcare professionals. The "evolution" of cancer.gov, and the NCI Facebook, Twitter, and YouTube networks are all projects that his creative team took from concept through launch. Previously, Roger spent 12 years as an award-winning Creative Director / Vice President at Walt Disney Imagineering where he had the opportunity to lead the creative development for a broad portfolio of projects ranging from PlayStation® games to theme park icons and several Disney World Celebrations; from mass audience interactive experiences and rides, to the MMOG Virtual Magic Kingdom. In "classic media," Roger has written and directed feature films and television, but is genuinely proud of researching and writing "The Living Sea" (Academy Award nomination for best documentary – Imax). Personally, Roger is a proud father; a 14+ year cancer survivor; and a competitive triathlete (3 events yearly), using the sport to raise research dollars for causes he supports.

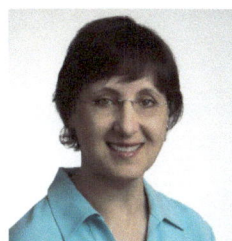

Adele Sender - Adele has developed clinical systems for healthcare software for complex chemotherapy regimens for diseases including HIV/AIDS and leukemia, and designed training modules for technology resource-poor environments as well as expert systems. She has a BS in Physical Therapy, and serves on both education and patient advocacy boards.

If you or someone you love has been diagnosed with a life threatening illness, Reimagine Well's Learn Guides are designed to guide you from diagnosis to wellbeing. We also provide a (private and safe) support community to connect with, where you can learn from the survivors and caregivers who have gone before you.

To learn more about our services, or to contact us directly, visit www.reimaginewell.com

www.ingramcontent.com/pod-product-compliance
Lightning Source LLC
Chambersburg PA
CBHW060801270326
41926CB00002B/51